Wakefield Press

Lifelines

Peter Couche lives in Adelaide with his wife, Simona. He has three adult daughters, Rebecca, Sarah and Sophie.

Lifelines

Breaking Out of Locked-In Syndrome

Peter Couche

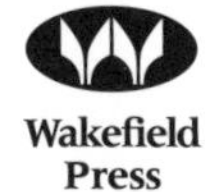

Wakefield
Press

Wakefield Press
1 The Parade West
Kent Town
South Australia 5067
www.wakefieldpress.com.au

First published 2007

Edited by Julia Beaven
Cover designed by Liz Nicholson, designBITE
Text designed and typeset by Clinton Ellicott, Wakefield Press
Printed and bound by Hyde Park Press, Adelaide

National Library of Australia
Cataloguing-in-publication entry

Couche, Peter (Peter Grant), 1950– .
Lifelines: breaking out of locked-in syndrome.

ISBN 978 1 86254 767 4 (pbk.).

1. Couche, Peter (Peter Grant), 1950– . 2. Cerebrovascular disease – Patients – South Australia – Biography. I. Title.

616.810092

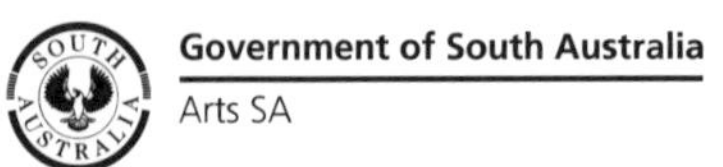

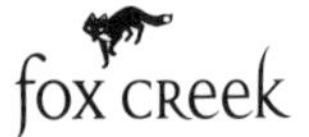

To my darling Simona, without whose constant care, love, and attention, this book may never have been written.

Contents

Foreword

Strokes are generally caused by an acute accident such as haemorrhage, thrombosis or embolism occurring in a weakened or diseased blood vessel responsible for supplying blood to the brain. Once the blood supply is cut off, the neurons (brain cells) in that part of the brain die, creating a permanent area of brain lesion (inactive cells).

The stroke Peter Couche suffered in February 1992 was no ordinary one. Called variously a brain-stem stroke or pontine infarction, it occurs in that section of the brain called the pons. The pons is part of the brain stem, which links the higher areas of the brain, the cerebral cortex, to the spinal cord and hence to the rest of the body. Thus a pontine stroke and infarction, if survived, is likely to result in a profound disconnection between the conscious mind and the rest of the body, inasmuch as no voluntary movement (facial expression, speech, gesture, posture, walking etc.) is possible.

The death rate when Peter suffered a pontine infarction was around 60 per cent, with most sufferers dying within the first four months. (Medical management has since improved and survival rates are now reported as high as 85 per cent.) The condition is believed to be irreversible; there is no treatment and no cure, and only sporadic reports in the medical literature of partial recovery. Research on the condition is quite sparse.

Typically, and in Peter's case, the result of a pontine infarction is loss of all physical functions – paralysis of all limbs and trunk, and loss of the ability to speak. Full mental comprehension is generally preserved, but while the person is aware of the external and internal environment, he or she is unable to communicate or interact with the world by word or gesture. The sufferer then becomes virtually an intact mind locked within a paralysed body, and for this reason the condition is often called 'locked-in syndrome'.

Usually, and again in Peter's case, there is preservation of an up-down movement of the eyes and movement of the upper eyelid. This makes a 'yes/no' form of communication possible, and words and sentences can be generated using an alphabet board, with Peter signalling with a movement of his eyes when the desired letter has been spoken by another person.

Peter also has some movement of his right forefinger, enabling him to operate a switch connected to a computer, by which means he is able to generate typewritten communications. The difficulties in communicating in this way are simply staggering. For example, each letter of the alphabet may require three or more presses of the switch, and take nearly a minute. A short paragraph of writing can therefore take hours and, because of the vagaries of the software or printer or involuntary pressing of the switch, sections can easily be inadvertently erased or lost – a demoralising experience.

Peter's use of the computer is also limited by a visual problem which makes it impossible for him to read normal-sized print from the screen. His electronic communication programme uses double-sized letters, and because the upper half of the screen is taken up by a menu grid, this leaves only a very small workspace for writing text. To write the early chapters of this book was relatively easy considering the obstacles involved, but the rewriting and editing was made well-near impossible by Peter's inability to read the original draft on his computer screen and revise it using a conventional word processing programme.

Nevertheless, in 1995, it was managed, with Carmel reading short sections of the draft out loud to Peter, suggesting changes or expansions, and relying on Peter's memory of what was required to amend the original draft.

Later work on the book was made easier by advances in technology and further progress in Peter's hand function. By 2006, Peter could use his index finger and the Words Plus computer programme to relatively quickly add details to the original draft notes to clarify and update the story. As Peter's amazing story unfolded, each draft was edited and returned for his approval and clarification, and then edited again. It took 13 years for the book to be completed.

For Peter to generate ordinary everyday communications and messages to family is an arduous and tedious process. To attempt to write a book is clearly a labour of Herculean proportions. The fact that this book was completed is testament to Peter's patience, courage and tenacity in the face of almost overwhelming difficulties. It is also an act of sheer defiance and unwavering determination to break out of his world of silence and have his extraordinary story heard.

Julia Beaven, editor
Carmel Tapping, psychologist

Prologue

I am sitting in my office, dressed in everyday clothes, and have a sense of urgency about what I am doing because my dear wife, Simona, will be here in less than two hours to collect me and take me home where I can sit outside in my garden.

It is important to set out these details, because they are in such marked contrast to the sterile, hospital-like institution where I spent more than six long years. There, patients wore either a tracksuit and runners (a touch of irony, what?) or a dressing gown and slippers – for the entire day. There, I would watch the slow progress of the clock hoping for a speedy end to another day. Now 24 hours is not enough.

In the institution I was marshalled into a daily routine

convenient to the staff, which only coincidentally suited me. Now, I pretty much do as I please. I draw up my timetable for allocation of time between work duties and the essential physical exercise my body needs in order for me to stay healthy and mentally alert.

There, I watched daytime television, and without a plan or a hope of leaving, my brain started slowly turning to mush. Around me patients grew institutionalised, devoid of individual character or will and therefore incapable of breaking free of the system.

Fortunately, while lying dormant in that institution, I grew to realise my brain was growing flabby and ineffectual due to lack of stimulation; hours of lying inert became opportunities for mental drills. What was that person's name from primary school who drove the teachers mad? I knew the answer was buried somewhere in my subconscious, all I had to do was find it. Or I multiplied 467 by 328 in my head, or named the Seven Wonders of the World.

With almost all physical functions denied me, I realised I had to rely on my mental capacity. This would be of crucial importance if I were not to become a be-slippered slobbering idiot, but instead be able to plan a way out of the institution in which I was trapped, and recapture my life.

This book is my story. In it I try to assess some of the factors which I believe contributed to my stroke, such a catastrophic physical event, and how I have tried to come to terms with its consequences. Like Icarus, I tried to fly too high and certainly too soon. I attempted in one generation to do what normally might take several – to move from rags to riches – for I was determined that my family would have only the best. I was to be the arch-provider and that, above all, required money and long hours of hard work.

My hope in writing this story is that it will serve as a warning for other people who are striving relentlessly for the trappings of material success. I hope it will cause them to take stock of their lives and ambitions, and to give thought to their long-term health and the wellbeing of their families.

But I hope also to increase the understanding of medical professionals and ordinary people of the difficulties, limitations and frustrations in daily living encountered by those whose lives have been constrained by severe disability.

This is not a fairy story, these are simple facts, achieved largely from the strongly held conviction that life is best lived by aiming at what is possible, not what is probable.

Chapter 1

Adelaide

Were you one of those children who ran everywhere instead of walking? I was. Perhaps the running symbolised the desire to have everything done yesterday.

I remember my grandfather's oft-repeated truism: top hats, bowyangs*, top hats. This saying is a cautionary one about discipline and ambition – the tendency of a family, over several generations, to move from relative wealth (and the hard work and discipline it took to get there) to relative complacency and a return to the bowyangs, until one of the bowyangs class decides, through hard work and discipline,

* Bowyangs: leather thongs used by poor folk to keep the legs of their trousers tight around the ankles to prevent mice, snakes, etc. from running up their legs.

to achieve top-hat status once again. I was determined never to be one of the bowyangs.

I am now convinced that these beliefs about the value of hard work and the quest for material success contribute to a continual state of stress, one of the major contributors to a stroke. Like the dripping of water on a stone, constant stress is corrosive.

Having always been aware of the connection between hard work and heart attack, I had taken care to keep myself fit – not that keeping fit was ever a chore because I really enjoyed it, especially running. About strokes, however, I knew absolutely nothing. I never made the connection between hard work and strokes and had no idea of what they were or how completely debilitating they could be. In my case, a stroke transformed my life overnight – from a promising career in a prestigious stockbroking firm to life as a severely disabled person, a quadriplegic, without the power of speech, and with the ability to move only my eyes and my right forefinger.

I was born into the relative post-war austerity of 1950 and attended Nailsworth Primary School, a co-ed State school whose main claim to fame was that bank robbers had once holed up there, and in the ensuing shoot-out with the police, bullets had entered the masonry. We didn't doubt this drama;

the bullet holes were still visible. At the age of eight I began piano lessons, thanks primarily to the determination of my mother, and every year for the next eight years there was an examination at the Conservatory of Music with a written exam in the theory of music. For an additional two years I studied Modern Music (rather than Classical), and became a devotee of boogie – which I remain to this day.

I progressed to Pulteney Grammar School, thanks again mainly to the persistence of my mother, a wonderfully forthright and affectionate woman, and clearly the daughter of her mother Ivy, both of whom I adore. In my second year at Pulteney I won an inter-school hurdles race and because it was something I was good at, and it enhanced my prestige with my school mates, I began to concentrate on it. Athletics – in fact all sport – and keeping fit and healthy quickly became an obsession. I weight trained relentlessly, ran and swam great distances, ate only fitness food (which presented something of a problem once the booze came along), and attended numerous holiday training camps.

Determination and self discipline became a way of life, and this has remained with me throughout my life, sustaining and driving me during the challenges of the last years.

I believe the most important three things in forming character are love, education and self-discipline. I firmly believe that each person, particularly in those formative early years, should work towards becoming as self-sufficient as possible. This means acquiring skills and pursuing knowledge at every level, and aspiring to be physically as well as mentally fit. And to be aware of, and be able to resist, the potentially dangerous and swerving influences of peers: risk-taking, the power of fashion, experimentation with alcohol, and sex. To counter the force of these influences I would set myself tasks, like running an extra lap at training, or having a cold shower in the morning.

At Pulteney Grammar I approached study and sport with equal intensity. I was, at best, only a moderate student, but the prevailing ethic at home was Calvinistic, so I tended to compensate for my lack of talent with pure slogging. In the field of sport I did hold some advantage – particularly athletics (ironic in light of subsequent events) – and later in swimming.

But I was my own worst enemy. As a young bloke I had a great passion for Australian Rules football as well as athletics. Football was my first choice, but fate had other plans and I turned out to be a reasonable athlete instead. My greatest enemy was never a fellow competitor, but always myself, one muscle pulling against another out of sheer tension.

As a Pulteney Grammar student, I played a football match against a Prince Alfred College team. I had leaped high for a

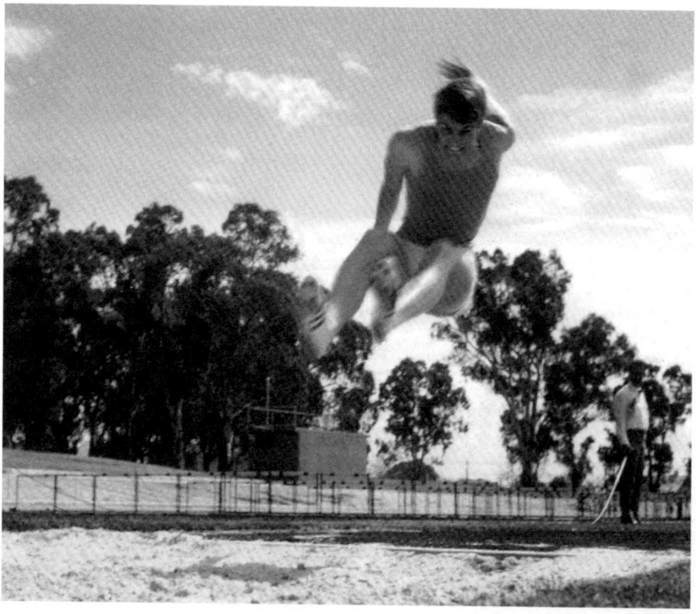

Competing in long jump at Kensington sports field, Adelaide, 1967

spectacular mark near the boundary and the cheering parents. Marking came easily to me because it was spur-of-the-moment stuff. I stepped back towards the crowd to take my set kick but managed only to kick the ball high into the air gaining no distance and fell flat on my bum in the attempt. I wished then that the ground would swallow me up. Here was an example of the difference between the relative ease I felt when performing spontaneously and the pressures of attention and too much time.

My father was the most intelligent man I have known. I have many memories of him, most of which are now dulled with time. But the overwhelming memory is of wisdom and kindness. I don't want this to be a defining description of my father, but it is indicative of him. It was a Saturday morning and I was in the Royal Adelaide Hospital (RAH) recovering from another battle with pneumonia. Hospitals are always ghastly, desolate places on weekends and my father had come to visit – which he always did no matter where I was. There I was lost in my thoughts, when who should stride in jauntily (pork-pie hat on his head, and carrying the paper) but my father, brightening the place considerably for me.

Toward the end of my time writing this book, my father passed away. I will never forget him saying to me when I was particularly affected by the all-encompassing awfulness of this bloody stroke that 'the sun will rise again one day'. He believed that a medical cure for this terrible affliction was 'out there' somewhere, so I had better stick around.

Largely a victim of circumstance – a 'strange' set of parents, The Great Depression, and the Second World War – he nonetheless had the good sense to guide both my brother and I through university and beyond and I attended the University of Adelaide, to study for a Bachelor of Economics, majoring in Commerce. In my first year I entered and subsequently won, on handicap, the Henley-Grange swim-thru which was then, as it is today, a two-kilometre ocean swim between two jetties. Later that same year I entered the Tunarama Festival swim-thru at Port Lincoln (about 270 kilometres south of my then place of holiday employment, the steel-making city of Whyalla). This event involved a swim of almost a kilometre between two grain jetties. I reckoned I had a fair chance but I faced the challenge of being hospitalised at the time for a spinal manipulation. The solution seemed simple; I decided to discharge myself immediately following the procedure. I remember walking up and down the corridors of the hospital to work off the effect of the anaesthetic and being asked stentoriously by the on-duty Sister, 'And what do you think you are doing?' Determined to compete I left the hospital, met up with a mate, and he drove me to Port Lincoln. But my problems were not over. While warming up for the race I stubbed my toe on a rock and broke it (my toe that is). Still determined, I hobbled out along the jetty in great pain, swam and won the race and my mate and I drove back to Whyalla where I checked myself back into hospital.

After a day spent working in the dreary offices of the steelworks in Whyalla I relaxed by swimming for hours in the main shipping channel, repeatedly clambering up the ladder to a little platform near the top, and diving in again.

I have a strong friendship with my brother Steve who is the funniest man I know. He is also loyal, loving, generous and wise. While I was at university, two nurses invited Steve and me to a black-tie ball to be held in the vast expanse of the Regency Ballroom. This was my partner's first ball so she and her mother had meticulously planned every detail. Steve, who had been doing field work in the Adelaide Hills, offered to drive and his car, a 1959 FC Holden, was filthy with grime. On the back seat lay a kit bag, a toilet roll, some hay and an awful lot of dirt.

My partner, who had swathed herself in organza for the occasion, had invited her parents down to wave her off. We approached the car as Steve made space on the back seat. I can picture him now furiously throwing things in the boot, under the scowling stare of her parents. And then with Mummy and Daddy waving farewell at the door, my brother reversed straight into the front wall, bringing down the letterbox and a huge chunk of masonry. He cheerily waved to the now ashen-faced parents as he hopped out of the car to readjust the fallen masonry and we then departed for the ball.

I guess this was as unremarkable as any ball, until we were preparing to leave and Steve decided to affect a drunken collapse. This necessitated dragging him across the vast ballroom floor with his feet limply scuffing along the

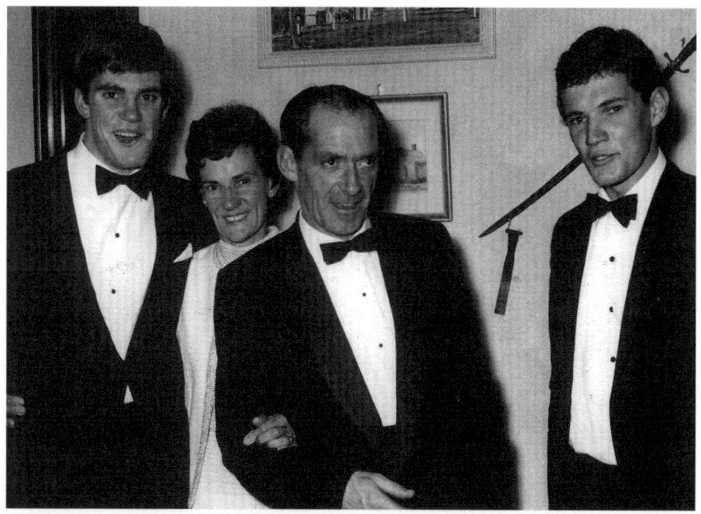

With my mother Lila, father Jack, and Stephen, at Stephen's twenty-first birthday, Adelaide 1969

floor behind. Needless to say, this attracted lots of attention. Miraculously, once outside, the cold night air seemed to completely restore him and we enjoyed a quiet and uneventful drive home. Perhaps, rightly, this was the high point of the girls' relationship with us.

This same girl (who deserved a medal for patience and forbearing) was also the subject of my attentions when I decided one day that it would be romantic to go rowing on the river. I had already chosen a relatively flat and grassy spot up-river, toward which we could head, and along the way I aimed to impress her with my rowing skills and charm. As we were rowing along, I decided that the coolest thing I could do (certain to impress I thought) would be to hoik a lurgy, macho-style, over the side as we were going along. Trouble was, instead of flying safely outside the boat and into the water it landed inside the boat and slid silently down one of the gunwales, probably covering her with spray as well. We rowed on in embarrassed silence.

At school I had won one of the first BHP Steel Industry Scholarships. In 1970 I attained my degree and it was time to leave my family and home in Adelaide and move to Melbourne to fulfil my commitment and commence employment with BHP, a big Australian mining company.

Chapter 2

Melbourne

I was always an intense perfectionist at work. Australia was facing deregulation of financial institutions and Britain, stock market deregulation. 'Work smarter, not harder' would have been a wise maxim to follow but I was convinced that hard work was the key to success. My father had recognised this when he said to me: 'I hope you have a champagne income boy, because you certainly have champagne tastes.'

In Melbourne I was to take up a position with BHP where, in exchange for a relatively meagre allowance as a Steel Industry Scholarship holder while at university, I was obligated to work for the next couple of years. My immediate boss, Graham Stephenson, one of the kindest men I have ever met, came to the airport to meet me on that first trip.

After three years of intense study I hit the ground running in Melbourne. Not only was I free of the burden of study, but I was in a new city, a new house, a new job, indeed a new life, free of the restrictions of home. I was ready to play.

But I was, I gather, rather an unusual person. It seemed I was always trying to pack more action into each day than most people would find necessary, or comfortable. I remember, at first, being nervous about my job, then bored, then critical of what I thought were the essentially menial tasks being asked of me. The controller came to me one day, and told me that he had a vitally important, top-secret job for me after work. I was nearly bursting with excitement and anticipation, believing that at last my true worth had been recognised. Imagine my disappointment when he led me into a room containing about 30 piles of paper, necessary for the company's AGM the next day. My 'secret' task involved being locked in that room and moving around the table stapling the various pages together.

High-spirited impulsivity and the habit of doing things to excess characterised much of my young days. This did not augur well for a long and successful career with BHP. The head office was then, and perhaps remains, a very . . . well . . . staid place. No facial hair of any kind was tolerated, and if you really wanted to get on, then it was suggested that you wore a dark suit and shoes, a white shirt and charcoal tie.

I was already at a disadvantage. I owned only one white shirt, but it had French cuffs. I wore it so often that the left sleeve became detached from the body of the shirt. I reckoned I looked pretty swish in French cuffs, even better than in my orange and brown shirt, or the one with yellow and green stripes. God they must have looked awful! In order for the cuffs of my white shirt to still be worn, I had to rip off the sleeves, leaving the body of the shirt and the two cuffs around my wrists. (You will appreciate that I had to keep my jacket on at all times.) My secret went undiscovered until one particularly hot day, during which I had many good-natured calls from my colleagues to 'take that bloody jacket off'. I finally succumbed to their entreaties and all was revealed, amidst hoots of laughter.

I was not only a leader in fashion, I also fancied myself as management material. I suggested to the controller that instead of eating at morning tea, the staff should engage in morning exercises. This, I pointed out, would not only save on the cost of morning tea with its consumption of sausage rolls and cake, but would result in more motivated and alert staff. I had been recently inspired by a Japanese steel-mill article on the subject. I should have left it at that, but not to be deterred by his lack of enthusiasm I progressed to demonstrating the exercises that I felt would be appropriate.

Again and again I ran foul of the senior staff. One day, while climbing the fire-escape stairs, ostensibly to keep fit but more to relieve boredom, I was overcome by the urge to take a leak. Unfortunately it happened to be near the floor where the 'heavies' worked. Well, there I was just minding my own business in the executive toilet when who should walk in but the bloody chairman. My breezy 'Good morning' was met with stony silence. I don't know why he was so perturbed – his was probably bigger than mine anyway – but by the time I made it back to my floor the gossip had spread and I was called into my boss's office to be given a thorough roasting.

On yet another occasion I was called into my boss's office, this time because of my 'low work energy'. He had chosen an unfortunate day to admonish me about this because I had been out all the previous night. As his lecture droned on, I felt overwhelmed by drowsiness and my eyes began to close.

While in Melbourne I rented, together with three other former economics students from Adelaide, half a two-storey house in Monomeath Avenue, Toorak. The other half was rented by some pretty air hostesses, and a piano tutor and her son Stanley. One cold evening we were running a bit short of firewood, so we solved this by chopping up the landlord's ladder and burning it. When that fuel source ran out, we removed all the wooden-framed fly-screens and burned them as well. On another occasion we sat on our share of the back lawn watching, of all things, Stanley's underpants fluttering in the breeze. Of course we decided to set them alight, starting with the underside of the pouch. I can no longer remember why this seemed such a good idea.

I enjoyed friendships with Steve Officer, a fellow flatmate, and Rod Gibson, both of whom I knew from economics days at Adelaide University. Rod lived with his parents in South Yarra, and we both fancied the girls who lived in the flat across the road. After a boozy lunch at his dad's new pub, we decided that this was to be the day we would meet the girls.

Just outside Rod's parents' place, someone had abandoned a supermarket trolley. It now seemed clear that a novel way of introducing ourselves would be to push the trolley up to the girls' door with Roderick inside. I rang the doorbell with young Rod stuffed into the trolley, pissed, arms and legs akimbo, but then changed plans and nicked off to hide behind a pillar. The door opened and revealed to the girls a very inebriated young Roderick crammed into the trolley, virtually speechless, and grinning widely. The girls proved tolerant and after this rocky start, we all developed a friendship.

When it came to alcohol, we were slow learners. One Saturday, Rod and I had a few kicks of the footy and ran a few laps of St Kevin's oval, so by the time we arrived back at his parents' place we were quite thirsty. We drank seven large cans of Carlton United beer before dinner. Rod's father, who fancied himself as something of a chef, was cooking that evening. I think we began the meal with fish-head soup, and after a couple of good reds, Rod's father retired for the night, and Rod and I settled in to sample his supply of port – Galway Pipe I believe it was.

Of the few people to whom I've told this tale, even fewer believe it. Rod's old man had, over the years, carefully collected and nurtured seven bottles of port. It took Rod and I much less time to consume them. In the middle of a drunken soliloquy somewhere through the seventh bottle, I endeavoured to make a point to Rod, only to find he was no longer where he had been at the head of the table. I was a bit narked that he had gone off to bed in the middle of my story. In fact the poor bastard's chair had up-ended and there, lying fast asleep on the floor with arms outstretched, was the boy in question.

After my couple of years in Melbourne, I returned in 1973 to the University of Adelaide to study for a Master of Business Administration. It was mid-way through this period of study that I began to work for myself and my career in business began in earnest.

Chapter 3

Adelaide

I first met Carmen in 1973 and we were married in my old school chapel on 25 October 1975. In no great rush followed the children – Rebecca in 1977 and Sarah two years later, both while we were living at Henley Beach in Adelaide.

I remember the birth of Rebecca particularly clearly. I had recently bought a 1932 Morris Commercial ex-PMG truck, which had its own air conditioning in the form of a substantial hole in the floor, through which the road was clearly visible. In the days leading up to Rebecca's birth I carefully reversed the truck up the steep driveway in preparation for a speedy departure for the hospital, hoping that it would not need a jump start when the moment came. I then placed bricks in front of the rear wheels and went in for a scrub up and a beer. When the time did come, around midnight, Carmen woke me and down to the truck we went, bricks away, and we rolled down the driveway and the hilly street for a perfect start and a somewhat noisy and breezy ride to the hospital.

Carmen and I were short of cash because I was always ploughing money back into some business venture. I think I had starved Carmen of housekeeping for seven weeks when I got it into my head that the waters immediately offshore from our place were likely to prove bounteous to the well-prepared spear fisherman. So I ventured into my local sports store determined to get properly kitted out. After about an hour I emerged with flippers, mask, snorkel, and a shiny new six-foot stainless-steel hand spear. I had taken the afternoon off and happily made my way down to the beach in the sunshine, smelling the fish I was about to catch. On the sand sat Carmen minding infant Rebecca, resplendent in a blue bonnet with yellow trim.

Greeting them both with a cheery hello, I donned my new gear. I was puzzled by Carmen's stony silence as I proudly displayed my new equipment, not making the connection between the lack of housekeeping and my brand new spear-fishing gear. I plop-plop-plopped my way out to deeper water scaring away any self-respecting fish. It was quiet and cold and I had condensation building up on the inside of my mask. I figured that I could easily wipe it clean if I just let go of my expensive new hand spear and let it rest on the featureless, sandy sea floor about ten feet down. This I did, but with my mask wiped clear I could no longer see my spear. Perhaps a current had taken me away from the spot where I had left it, and perhaps once I had finished cleaning my mask, I had swum off in the wrong direction. Despite searching for a good half hour I was forced to admit defeat, and return to shore without the spear, or any fish.

While at the University of Adelaide I had recruited staff for a waiting service and met Guy – 'Fitz' – who was to become a life-long friend. Together we ran what was then known as the Weir Restaurant, as well as providing staff for many of the parties in town. Fitz was indispensable. I remember one evening at the Weir Restaurant, when all the staff and diners had left for the night and the theatre crowd was beginning to arrive. Fitz decided to put on his own floor show under the spotlights with his trousers rolled up. The audience was enthralled and showed no sign of ever going home. At dawn I told the theatre-goers that the restaurant was now closing and ordered them home to their beds.

The waiting business was inspired by my latter months in Melbourne, where I had found working as a part-time waiter in the evenings at private parties and functions a reasonably

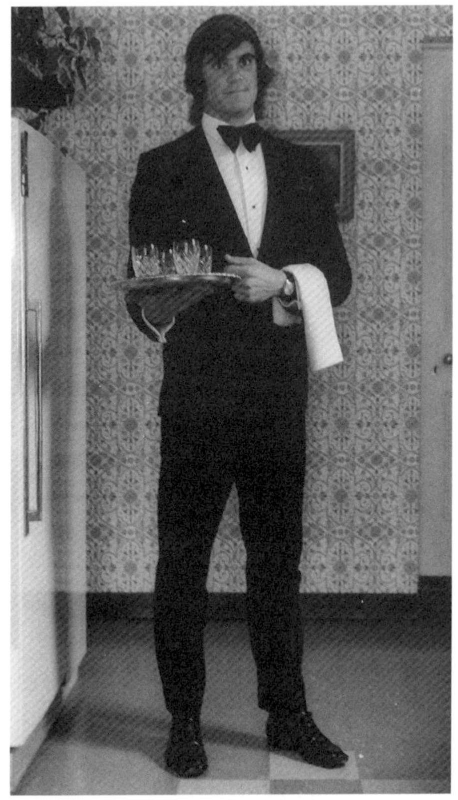

At work as a waiter, while running the Weir Restaurant, Adelaide, 1973

pleasant way to earn some cash. But the cost of using a hiring firm was high so I set one up and later bought an established party hire business, Hickox Hire, with a partner, John. It was a table-ware time warp – linen damask table-cloths and super-fine sherry glasses – but it was a good buy. The idea was that John would put up the money and I would run the business. We would then split the profits half and half. I remember we sold the front block of land for more than the price of the entire business. This, plus the fact that we trusted each other, made the thing work. But God, it was hard going! In vertically integrating Hickox, we also moved into the wine business, becoming a sales outlet for a now defunct winery. Apart from having awful wine, this particular company came up with the brilliant strategy of marketing sweet and dry sherry by putting the same product in identical bottles but with a different label on each. That would keep the punters guessing.

Unfortunately this grand strategy came unstuck when, at a wedding reception, I offered a grand old dame the choice of a sweet or a dry sherry – they were all sweet on my tray of course. Well, she opted for dry and I proceeded to the bar to get that which I didn't have and promptly returned with yet another glass of the same brown viscous liquid and a hatful of profound apologies. In return, she roundly abused both me and the brown viscous liquid, and one could hardly blame her. Soon after we parted company with this enterprising organisation.

We employed a young man named Jimmy. One morning young James and I embarked in the brand new Holden utility emblazoned with HICKOX plus a very old trailer to pick up a dance floor we had put down the night before. It was raining heavily when we began loading the floor onto the old trailer. This made the downhill slope into the place an altogether different proposition when leaving. We loaded the dance floor on to the trailer, tied the pieces down, and somehow or other got up the slope. But our troubles were only just beginning.

We hadn't travelled far before the smell of burning rubber indicated that the weight of the dance floor on the axle had pushed the mudguards onto the tyres. The solution was simple: pull into a service station, borrow a set of bolt cutters and cut off the mudguards. Of greater concern were the rumblings which were beginning to be emitted from James – something about the work being too 'effing' hard and the 'effing' weather.

Admittedly it was now beginning to pour, and I was probably ten years or more his junior. We set off in the driving rain down the freeway, only to find that the tread on the outside tyre had worn loose due to the rubbing of the mudguards. Sure enough, a short distance later we lost that tyre and replaced it with the spare from the new utility.

We now had a trailer with different sized wheels and a heavy dance floor on top. We made it to within 600 metres of the yard before the entire wheel came off and the chassis of the trailer buried itself deep into Unley Road. This was at the time of the introduction of the new clearway system, so there were plenty of police about. I explained my dilemma to one of them and was smartly told to get moving or we would get a ticket when the clearway restrictions came into effect ten minutes later. Even James was galvanised into action by that.

While I borrowed a heavy-duty jack from a nearby service station, young James nicked into the local hardware store and brought back six mild steel bolts, which was all they had. Hastily, we jacked up the trailer and replaced the sheared off hard steel studs with the mild steel ones. We made it within the time limit and limped back to the yard, leaving behind only the gouge we took out of Unley Road. Once back in the yard, the trailer gave up the ghost completely and the wheel literally fell off. That expression has amused me ever since. Although James declared it an 'effing' awful day, I think we escaped rather lightly.

The waiting business and the party hire business were thriving but it was impossible to run both so in 1975 the waiting business was sold. This should have left me to concentrate my energies on party hire, but instead I immediately expanded into construction hire. Responding to an advertisement in the paper, I visited this rather strange and sad man and we hit it off to the point where I bought his business on the spot. John's reaction later that day was not so much 'good on you' as 'good God!' – I was only supposed to look at the business, not buy the bloody thing!

Anyone can tell you the folly of mixing two different hiring businesses and, although Hickox Hire had also thrived, it was sold to the competition. John left amicably and I was left to build up construction hire. I did this in two ways. First, I created a company shell called Savage Construction Hire and bought second-hand builders' equipment and hired it out, and I purchased a tired old business, Multiple Form Constructions Pty Ltd. We were swamped by business related to the national building boom. Second, I bought new equipment, leased new trucks, employed six staff and secured the lease of the adjoining back block. This more than quadrupled our land size and allowed vital rear access. I was ably assisted by my super secretary (my mother) as well as by ex-teacher and later family friend, Mike B. The business prospered aided by another Mike, who used to keep fit by running in from Morphett Vale to the business on Whittam Street (a distance of about 25 kilometres) with a house brick in each hand.

We also employed an accident-prone chap by the name of Rolf. When I asked him to burn some rubbish he set fire to the bloody fence as well. After a bit of a panic during which the burning fence was extinguished and the neighbours placated, I thought it only fair to let him try again. But he managed to do it all over again – fence and all. The final straw came one Friday night when Rolf returned to the yard with the superstructure of the brand new trailer at a precarious angle. It later transpired that he had reversed straight into a tree, but at the time all he was capable of saying was 'it wasn't my fault' over and over again. Endlessly interesting though Rolf made our lives, we just couldn't afford to keep him, and we paid him off that night.

Good fortune was surely on my side when I was driving to work one Saturday morning in the new 15-foot tray-top with the new trenching machine trailer on the back. I made a right turn into Unley Road, whereupon my own trailer passed me on the right-hand side. Damn, I thought, I've forgotten to put on the safety-chains. My unladen heavy-duty steel trailer was heading off down Unley Road with me in hot pursuit, its nose into the centre of the road causing sparks to fly, and cars darting to the left and right to get out of the way of the bloody thing. The chap who owned the plumbing shop was standing near a street sign, trying to see what all the noise was about. The trailer by this stage had moved over to his side of the road and was heading his way. It neatly mounted the kerb in front of him, decapitating the street sign. Then it turned left, straight into a used tyre yard and a pile of used tyres. No real damage was done to either people or vehicles, though God knows how. Thoroughly chastened I picked up the trailer and quietly headed back to my yard.

In building up Savage, we exploited two niches in the market. One was the market for foundation boards – boards used in constructing the foundations for houses – and no one else in Adelaide, or perhaps even in South Australia, did this. Secondly, we hired out templates for archways. I had spotted houses being built down south with archways for architectural decoration. This was a natural for a hiring situation. I found it appealing to own something, hire it out and then get it back again. So long as the equipment was maintained the return on investment was fantastic.

Why sell the business, you may ask, if it was that good? Well, no one ever went broke making a profit and the moral remains: always leave something for the other guy and get out while the going is good. Savage Hire was probably the highlight of my working career and I often look back on it wistfully.

By then I had worked out a grid system for any new business. There were two hard and fast rules: don't become involved in any business which has high inputs and a large staff but, more importantly, don't become involved with a business where seasonality (i.e. spoiling or fashionability of output) is a big factor.

In 1977 I bought Adelaide Bin and Pallet with Mike B who I had worked with for years in the hiring business. Bin and Pallet fitted the grid perfectly as it consisted of one big shed for sawing and one for making pallets and bins. There was an office attached (or at least a separate room) containing a table, a chair, a working phone, and a working dunny. Neither Mike nor I had any experience in this area but figured (correctly as it turned out) that there was enough slack in the business to allow us to learn from our mistakes. And there were plenty of those in the early days. To begin with I worked until early afternoon preparing the hiring business for sale (so many memories, so much work) and then until early evening at the pallet place.

When we bought the business, the 'making' shed was full of off-cuts from a previous owner. We worked like navvies to get that shed clear and the business on a sound footing. By one means or another, I had become chief sawyer which meant, among other things, working in front of a 30-foot circular band saw all day. One day I was working away in front of the saw with my face pressed hard against a log, when out from the bark crawled a bloody great centipede which attempted to make its way up my nose. This was dirty, dangerous, frightening, exhausting, and extremely noisy work. Each morning when I started the band saw I wondered if I would lose any fingers that day.

The space between the sheds was filled with the company's only primary input, logs from a government log licence. Situated as it was near the city dump and many of the local tanneries – in an era before noise, smell or other pollution controls – it was far from pleasant when there was a hot north-westerly blowing or even worse, a dust storm from the west.

We worked hard, the business grew and we employed around five Vietnamese refugees. But both Mike and I were looking for a safer, quieter, less stressful existence. In 1979, after about two years, we payed off our debts, pocketed a few bob, and tidied the business for sale. When we were approached with an offer to buy, we grabbed it.

At about this time, Carmen and I decided to buy a run-down cottage in the city, the idea being that we would buy the place, renovate and let it, and then use the profits to buy another one. I cannot remember a more peaceful time than this, yet we decided to move to Sydney because of the lure of the Sydney surf. By the time we left for Sydney we had two very young children and seven very old cottages.

Chapter 4

Sydney

When we arrived in Sydney, there were no job prospects in hand, but my great mate Rod had at least given me the name of a fellow who worked for a broking house. So I took this chap out for lunch and discovered that he had hollow legs. The lunch had been organised to ensure that I had a broking contact while in Sydney so that I could continue my share transactions. We then proceeded on to dinner. The point of all this (apart from the amount of booze consumed, which was prodigious) was that I eventually met Mr Brian C France, then head of Meares & Philips, and one of the finest men I was ever to meet.

And so it came about that with a wife and two tiny children to care for, I joined a broking house. I reckoned that compared to anything else I had done, broking had to be easy. I was soon to learn that being a good broker was just the opposite.

We bought a small terrace house (although we thought it was huge) in Windsor Street, Paddington. As we signed the deal, I reckon there was a bloke standing outside with a bloody great gong which he struck to signal the end of the real-estate boom. At the same time, shares of both of my companies were suspended from trading and the market crashed – with me locked in, or, rather, out. That little exercise cost me about $100,000. That very night I resolved to be the best damned broker that Meares had ever had.

By working hard during the day and studying at night, I successfully completed the AISCA course and within two years I had been admitted to the partnership assisted, no doubt, by the lobbying of my two friends Brian France and Tim Crammond.

Shortly after being admitted to the partnership, the question of a car arose, and it was suggested that the partnership buy a new car which I could then lease back from them. The trouble was that I neither wanted nor needed a new car, being perfectly happy with the one I had – an old Jaguar XJ6. I proposed to the firm that instead of going to all the trouble of buying a new car, why not just buy my old one from me and have me lease it back from the firm instead. This way I would get to keep the car I wanted.

The very night this transaction was finalised (with me waxing lyrical to Carmen about our new-found financial security over dinner), some bastard tried to pinch the car. Lying in bed that night I was awakened by familiar coughing and wheezing sounds. I thought vaguely 'that sounds like our car'. Then, suddenly awake, I thought 'that bloody well is our car'. I raced downstairs in time to see the firm's latest asset disappearing down the street.

I rang the police and explained that if they were quick, they should be able to catch the thief before he escaped the intricate streets of Paddington.

But even while this conversation was being conducted I heard the familiar wheezing sounds again, and despite all the front lights in the house now blazing, found that whoever had taken the car had not only brought it back but was trying to park it as well!

I hung up on the police, determined to belt the thief first and maybe ask questions later. However, when I opened the car door I was greeted by a person who was obviously a total simpleton. After letting him go, it just remained to await the arrival of the police.

When they finally arrived it was about 4 am, and I was asked questions such as: 'Now which window were you looking out of when you first noticed the car missing?' and, 'Which window were you looking out when you noticed it had returned?' In addition to the police thinking that they must have a right one here, they obviously also thought I was shickered.

I discovered that young 'Jack Brabham' was on some sort of roving brief to nick classic or semi-classic cars, but when he had taken mine to the meeting point, he must have been told to take the heap of crap back where he had found it. And that is exactly what he had done. Bloody hell! I must be one of the few people to have a car stolen and then returned, neatly parked.

In relation to that very same car, I received a phone call from Carmen at work one day, enquiring quietly, in the middle of a busy dealing session, whether we had fire insurance on the car. I replied that we hadn't, and then of course thought that was a funny question for her to ask. I learned that Carmen had headed off with the girls in the back when the engine had exploded into flames from petrol leaking out of a faulty carburettor onto the engine block. After she and the children had escaped and the fire brigade had been called to put out the blaze, she had phoned me.

I then committed the cardinal error of not only neglecting to ask after her and the children immediately, but also of wondering out loud why, since the insurance on the car was worth more than the car itself, she had bothered to turn the engine off, thus preventing completion of the job.

To burn off excess energy, apart from walking four or five kilometres to and from work, I ripped up the back yard. Since it consisted of concrete over asphalt over concrete over asphalt, I hired a jack-hammer and got started. By the time I had finished, after many late night visits to a local building site to dump concrete rubble, we had a reasonable brick-paved back yard laid out with railway sleepers and ferns. We had the children set their feet and hand prints in wet concrete and dated it 11/82.

At work I was learning that there were different kinds of stress. Running a sawmill and getting lots of exercise was very different to sitting motionless at a desk all day. Since my early twenties I had been experiencing distressing symptoms that would typically last 24 to 48 hours. The pattern never seemed to change. I suffered nausea, vomiting, headaches and pain throughout my body, and often lost consciousness for brief periods, perhaps a couple of minutes. Fortunately, I suffered no resulting neurological deficits such as slurring of speech or loss of limb function. Visits to doctors did little good. By the time I got there the symptoms had usually passed, and my visits generally only resulted in a warning to slow down.

We enjoyed Sydney and met many fine people there including the Wenhams, the Raines and the Krantzes. My shares had since been re-listed for trading and were quickly sold. Life was good. In March 1983 Tim Crammond, the institutional partner heading our desk, invited me to lunch at the Australia Club and said, over dessert, 'Well, someone has to go and fix up London, and it ain't gonna be me!' There was little doubt that the London office needed a boost, with staff morale, revenue and client numbers low, but leaving Sydney was a real wrench.

Chapter 5

London

We hit London running. At that time broking was still in its infancy. I remember beginning at Warnford Court for Meares & Philips, where we not only had to share a key for the men's loo way down the end of the passage, but we had no running water. In 1982/83 financial markets were deregulated and Meares & Philips was taken over by Barclays. I worked very hard as a broker, and in our new building, complete with the luxury of an easily accessible loo, I set about putting together a fine young team spearheaded by the redoubtable, ever-reliable Andrew J Crichton, ably assisted by Charlie R D Wittenoom and Rodney J Walker.

The square mile of London, known as the City or the financial district, was completely foreign to me when I first arrived. Like a square peg in a round hole, I found cold and grey old London very different from the sunny Sydney town to which I had become accustomed. I can even remember office workers stripped down to what they delightfully called a vest (singlet) at their appointed lunch break, spread out on the grass, soaking up the available sunshine – at the end of which they would put their shirts back on and return to work.

This was the most stressful period of my working life. Working all day in front of a 30-foot band-saw wasn't exactly peaceful and stress-free, but I could at least work off tension with hard, sweaty, physical exercise. This was in marked contrast to the world in which I now found myself, a place in which success was measured, among other things, by one's skill with the telephone.

The stage was now set for my final descent into, and ultimate emergence from, a devastating stroke.

I had learned very little regarding working 'smarter not harder' because I worked harder at that time than at any other, gaining a foothold in the London stockbroking market. Of course I should have relaxed more, taken everything slower and easier, and submitted myself to far less stress – but that was not my way at the time.

Our task was to broke Australian stocks to British and European institutions, and to keep the order flow as high and as consistent as possible. Thus, there was pressure to perform every day, every week, every month. This is not the full story, but I can say with some certainty that I would be happy to pursue my goals with the workmates I then had at my side. We were a good team and we managed to make some headway, and the number of clients with whom we did business began to grow.

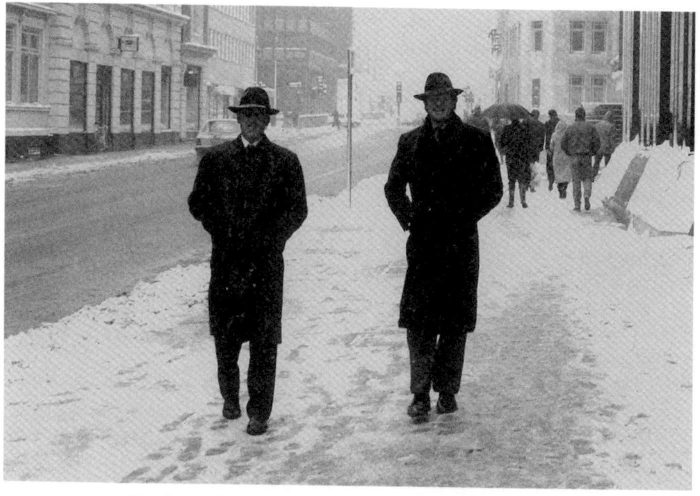

With Andrew Crichton, London, winter 1989

London was kind to us. We began by renting a house for two years in Lamont Road, Chelsea (or World's End to be more precise). On our first Guy Fawkes' night in London I decided to have a little fireworks display, but it seemed that I bought enough crackers for the entire street. On a freezing evening, our little group assembled in our pocket handkerchief-sized back yard to watch me try to become a household name in pyromania.

I had sky rockets as long as my arm and bungers that could compete with a hand grenade. I was not in familiar territory, but armed with the tolerance of the neighbours, we sallied forth.

After an hour or two we crept back inside, half scared out of our wits, and without letting off even half the fireworks I had bought. I subsequently discovered that our evening had been spent breaking the law, fireworks being permitted only in public places. On the same night a display was held for the public just down the road in Battersea Park.

On our corner of Lamont Road lived David Browne, his wife Fruma and their two boys. David took the time to introduce us to London, and to innumerable bottles of excellent champagne. Whether it was the Royal Automobile Club, the Racing Club, the Derby, Jermyn Street, Simpson's, or Jacko's, David would be there to introduce us or squire us through.

Jacko's was unique. It was listed in the phone book under a quite different name. The restaurant specialised in revolting food prepared by Jacko's good wife Shirl, whose 'double, double, toil and trouble' mien reminded us of Macbeth's witches straight in from the heath. The food was served by the irrepressible Pearl who, if you were really on his good side, greeted you with a couple of kisses, and wine every bit as revolting as the food. Despite the lousy food and wine, I can scarcely remember relaxing more at a restaurant than at Jacko's.

The walls, ceiling and every nook and cranny were filled to overflowing with objets d'art, while the upstairs room, cordoned off, was smart and created an air of exclusivity. There Jacko Leech hung his paintings, and it seemed like we bought half our paintings from him. I remember one evening I was once again in the upstairs room viewing my favourite painting of the Thames at low tide (by a Royal Academician, also a Leech), when who should come up the stairs but Jacko, whose alleged favourite it was also, and who had consistently refused to sell it to me.

This particular night he finally wavered and we settled on a price of £2500. I suggested tossing a coin for the right to purchase, he agreed, and I proceeded to lose the first toss which left me £2500 down with no painting. Well, some three paintings and £6000 later I finally got him to sell. The next morning I rang him and we agreed that just the £2500 for the picture was fair exchange. Bloody good of him really, especially since I reckoned the painting was cheap at twice the price.

On another evening, the tail-end of a fancy-dress party

seemed to have gathered at Jacko's. That evening Carmen and I were seated near the front door when two girls entered, one wearing a dress that lifted her naked breasts as though on a shelf. I recall her nipples were like cherries. Perhaps she went as some kind of fruit salad. The other girl was clad in nothing but swathes of cling wrap. It was Bohemia at its best, and both Carmen and I loved it.

On yet another evening there, my friend Andy and I parted with 400 perfectly good pounds for the privilege of owning a heavy cruet set consisting of salt and pepper shakers in the shape of two very large gilt-bronze erect penises nestling in a little silvered tray. I was certainly not able to keep them at home, and I suspect Andy wasn't either. So we took the bloody thing to work and proceeded to award it in turn to whoever had done the last big deal, and to any visiting secretary who, for whatever reason, was considered fair game.

At this time Bonhams in London were conducting auctions in erotica, and after Andy and I had had our fun at the office, we offered the cruet set for sale. As he held it aloft, I can still hear the auctioneer saying, 'Well, this really takes the biscuit'. We didn't get our money back, but we'd had a ripper time with it in the meanwhile. The auctions in erotica were later discontinued, perhaps because of too much attention from the raincoat brigade.

I had always believed in what was possible, rather than probable. The day that I was due to fly back to London after a trip to Sydney dawned warm and clear, and I figured that before returning to the cold and the grime of London, one more swim in the surf of Sydney was in order. Trouble was, I didn't have a hire car and time was limited. But I figured by acting quickly with the help of a taxi I could possibly both swim and get to the airport on time to board my flight. So I packed up my things, checked out of my hotel and hailed a cab. I explained my predicament to the taxi driver and he seemed prepared to ferry me around to get it all done. This meant an initial stop at a store to buy (while the taxi driver waited) a towel and soap and then off to Bronte Beach for a much-anticipated swim. I could glimpse the driver, as I bobbed up and down in the swell, on the lawn, anxiously awaiting my return (but with the meter no doubt still ticking away). After my swim I showered, put my wet swimming togs into a little plastic bag I had brought along for that purpose, and walked out to the taxi for the trip to the airport and the 20-hour flight to London. I gave the soap and towel to the taxi driver with my thanks, and walked onto the plane carrying the little plastic bag.

In 1984, when my liver could stand it no longer, we left Lamont Road and bought a place in Lansdowne Road,

Notting Hill. This charming house was a wonderful place to bring up children, backing as it did onto several acres of communal garden and was just over the road from the generous and generally wonderful Mike and Suzy Schneideman, who became our close friends. And in 1988 came little Sophie to complete our family of beautiful girls.

Lansdowne Road was just a spit from the Portobello Market where we ventured on Saturday mornings, me sporting Sophie on my shoulders eating an ice cream (which would drip onto my head), with Rebecca and Sarah holding onto each hand, especially if there were boys about, as we scoured the markets for bargains. We would then indulge in Italian food for lunch, purchased from Mr Christian's: salami, rich cheese, Italian bread, tomatoes and fresh basil, washed down with lots of lovely white wine. After lunch, a quick 'silly walk' home which one of the big girls won – often Sarah.

At around this time I had one of those 'at least I did it' life experiences; I bought a boat, the *Sulara*. She was a genuine 1924 Camper and Nicholson, powered by twin Gardener 114 BHP diesels and measuring 103 feet from tip of bowsprit to stern. Rigged as an all-wooden schooner, she was beautiful. She slept five people comfortably, six at a pinch, and had two bathrooms, one with the pure Edwardian extravagance of a bath! She was permanently moored in Antibes on the French Riviera, playground of the rich and famous – trouble was, I was neither!

She was bought in a spirit of great optimism. I thought I could use her as a training ground to prove to myself that I could still run a small business, for she was to be the *Orient Express* of the Mediterranean, or so I thought. My enterprise managed to be promoted on magazine covers, in newspaper articles (including the *Weekend Financial Times*) and on television, and early on we secured sponsorship of the Carlton Intercontinental Hotel in Cannes.

But it was to little avail. It was 1990 and the boat was chartered out for £1500 per day – a ludicrous amount of money and too much for all but the wealthiest of people. Thus, charters were hard to come by and she was used instead for family holidays (which was, after all, why she was bought in the first place).

Despite this, for a time we moved in amazing circles. I was invited to the opening of the Carlton Intercontinental Casino, where the roulette table had chips for US$1million each. I also remember an extremely long red carpet being rolled out across the Croisette, the madly busy four-lane esplanade, and up the pier to the hotel's private jetty where the boat was moored. The family and I dutifully disembarked and strode on up to the hotel, between the topless

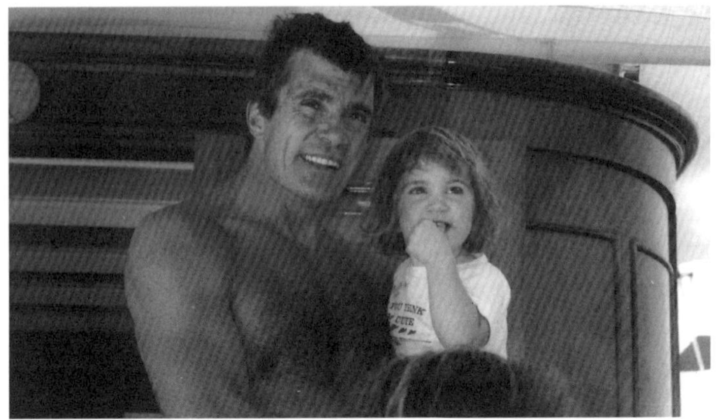

With Sophie on the deck of *Sulara*, French Riviera, 1990

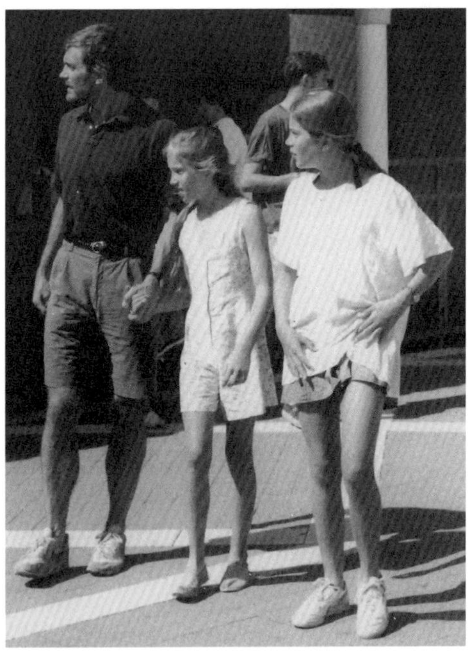

Shopping on the French Riviera with Sarah and Rebecca, summer 1990

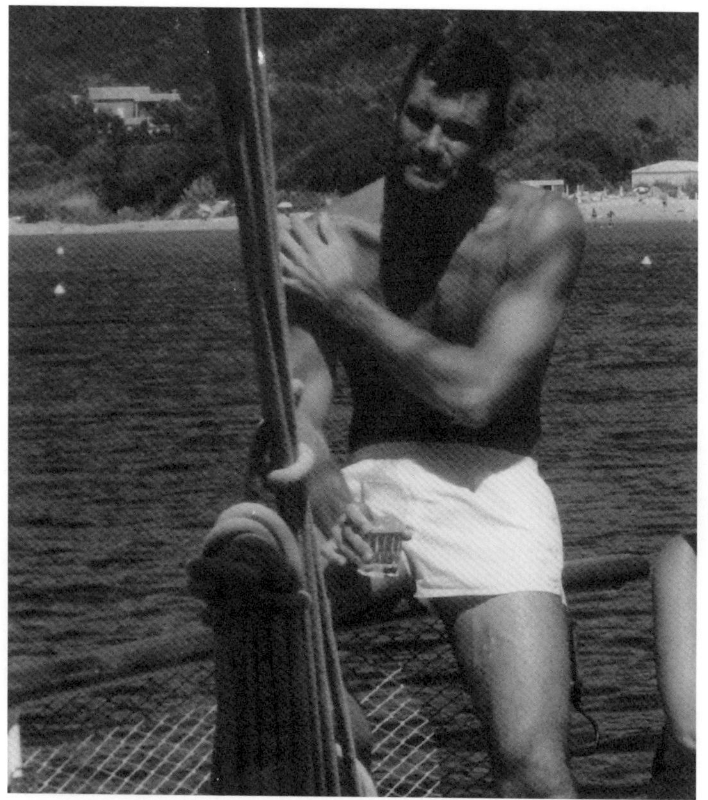

On holiday with my family sailing on *Sulara*, Antibes, France, summer 1990

blondes on either side of the pier, and a bevy of young starlets strategically laid out on the sand. I remember this incident because I was carrying a brown hold-all, made not of leather but of vinyl, and one of the handles had broken, so I had affected running repairs by tying the handle to the bag in a rather clumsy knot! I hope I just looked eccentric.

As a charter vessel *Sulara* was not ideal but for the family, especially Carmen, she became the perfect holiday vessel. We came to know the south of France and the north of Italy. The captain, chosen by me, was something of a disaster, and this added to my stress. I don't agree at all with the notion that owning a boat is like standing under a cold shower in a raincoat ripping up fivers – it's more like ripping up fifties!

As a family, we enjoyed some wonderful times on board that boat. One morning, I remember surfacing on deck, resplendent in my business suit and tie, whereupon I said my cheerio's to the family and hopped in a taxi for the Nice airport to catch a direct flight to London. A speedy taxi at the London end could see me to my office by late morning; one minute on board a boat in sunny France and the next, behind a desk in rainy London. (Once again giving proof to the theory that life was the art of the possible, not the probable.)

I found myself in the somewhat invidious position of working longer and more stressful hours (roughly 7 am to 7 pm) broking at all hours, usually behind a desk, looking after Carmen and the children, and operating the boat. My volume of work had therefore increased rather than decreased and in fact I was seeing even less of my family, which was completely defeating the purpose.

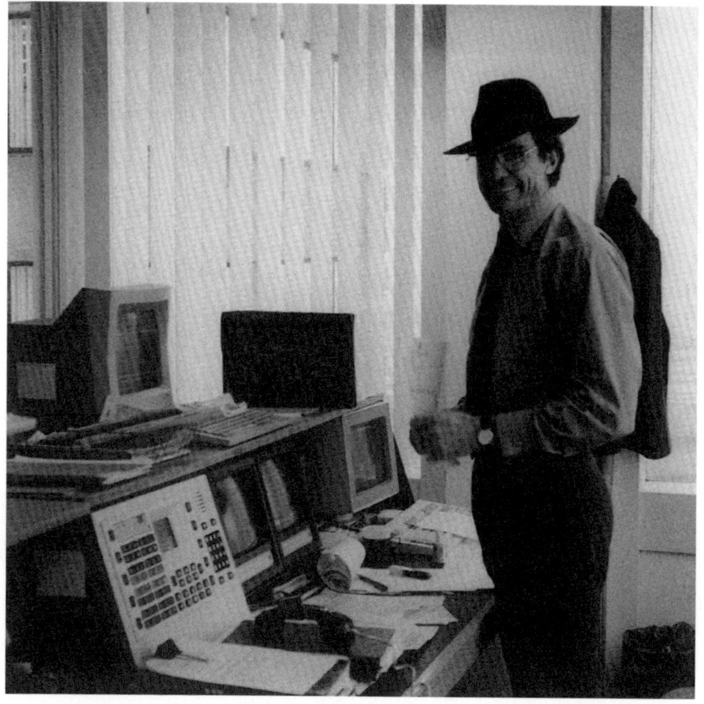

Back at work at BZW, stockbroking firm, London, 1990

And time was running out, although I did not realise it. I had been broking Australian stocks for nigh on ten years in London, and had just been offered the position of managing director of the Singapore office. Although clearly I was not seeing enough of Carmen and my three beautiful children, I nevertheless went out to Singapore not once but twice. I was confident I could turn the Singapore office around, but it would probably have killed me in the process, for what resulted from my last journey to Singapore was no ordinary attack of the usual symptoms. Little wonder really that I just blew up one day, like a perfectly good car which, having blown its carburettor, can no longer spark its moving parts into life.

Chapter 6

Singapore

In 1992 the family had holidayed in Western Australia and we had stopped off in Singapore on our way home to London. Carmen and the children had stayed with relatives while I checked into a hotel to attend to business.

My next visit to the island was a short while later, and was clearly a junket to celebrate the opening of the Bangkok office of Barclays, of which my stockbroking firm was a subsidiary. God knows the firm couldn't afford the celebration as our desk was not having a good month.

Walking about Singapore that February evening, I began to feel a little odd. I had already spent a couple of productive days at the office there and it was suddenly the weekend, and Valentine's Day in London, where I had organised gifts for

Carmen and the girls. I settled down to a room-service meal, complete with wine, in front of the television. Before turning in I phoned home and spoke to Sarah.

After a good night's sleep, I rang down for breakfast. A shower was in order but as I stepped into the shower and turned on the taps, I noticed that my left arm was shaking suddenly, violently, and then my left leg. At first I thought this was just another attack of the kind I was accustomed to. I stumbled from the shower and collapsed on the floor. Cancel breakfast, I remember thinking, I must cancel breakfast. Dry-retching I made it to the hall mirror, where a pale face stared back at me but try as I might, I couldn't make the extra few feet to the door to call for help. The long, long nightmare had begun.

I remember an ambulance being called, and lying on the bed dreading the thought – the bother of it. I didn't want to miss my friend Greg who lived in Singapore and had promised me a banana-leaf curry in the old part of town. But I waited, I had no choice, as an obese member of the hotel staff sat nearby reading my bloody newspaper.

I had never been in an ambulance before and it was a strange experience being carried out the back door of the hotel and into the waiting ambulance for the trip to Mount Elizabeth Hospital. I could still talk and swallow and I explained as best I could to the kind and patient nurse inside what had transpired. How we take things for granted!

I was placed under the care of Dr Tang. Extracts from my medical reports at that time trace the progress of my condition:

Mr. Couche is a 41-year-old stockbroker from the city of London who arrived in Singapore on 13 February 1992 via Bangkok. On the morning of 15 February 1992 he developed jerking of the left lower limb while in the shower. He experienced severe vertigo and had double vision. He tried to get out of the bathroom but fell because of severe unsteadiness ... He is married with children. He was described as a workaholic who worked very long hours and very intensely ...

... Alert and rational and could give a good history. Orientated to time, place and person ... moderately severe dysarthria. No dysphasia ... mild ptosis especially right side. Loss of lateral gaze ... impaired upgaze but preserved downgaze ... mild left lower motor neuron facial paresis ... severe truncal and appendicular ataxia. Severe inco-ordination in both upper limbs with gross dysmetria ... He was transferred to the Intensive Care Unit where a re-examination at 3 pm revealed further neurological deterioration.

At 3 pm his speech had become more severely dysarthric . . . He had developed paralysis of the left upper and lower limbs. Examination at this time revealed severe right ptosis with bilateral facial paresis . . . There was a dense left hemiplegia with both lower limbs going into frequent severe extensor spasms.

By 7 pm he had become anarthric and developed weakness of the right side with difficulty swallowing. At this time he could still signal by blinking twice to indicate 'yes' . . . His blood gases remained satisfactory but pulsed oximetry indicated progressive desaturation. This plus increasingly laboured breathing and excessive pharyngeal secretions necessitated endotracheal intubation and respiratory support at 5 am on the morning of Sunday 16 February.

By 8 pm on Sunday 16 February he had developed ocular bobbing but remained able to intermittently blink twice to commands. He continued to show signs of being aware of his environment . . . Clinically he has the locked-in syndrome . . . we remain hopeful that some degree of neurological recovery will occur . . .

Carmen and my brother Steve had both dropped everything and within 48 hours of my admission to the hospital Carmen arrived, followed by Steve. They stayed with my friend Greg and his family and were lent a car by my company. I was fortunate to be visited by both of them daily, and that stopped me worrying about my tardiness in returning to London. By then I had sunk beneath the inky blackness of speechlessness.

I have always felt that it was then, immediately after admission to hospital, that therapy should have commenced, including vigorous movement of my limbs. But that depended on a prompt and accurate diagnosis which did not occur in my case, principally because so little was known of my condition then. Instead I was kept completely immobile on a sweaty hospital bed – for weeks – during which time my feet collapsed and my muscles wasted, before I received any limb mobilisation or physiotherapy.

At first, it was thought I had multiple sclerosis or an unusual form of brain-stem encephalitis, since a brain scan had not revealed any signs of a lesion in the cerebral hemispheres or brain stem. But by then I knew that despite my physical fitness, too much work, too much booze and, above all, too much stress, are bad auguries for a stroke.

Eventually, a tentative diagnosis of brain-stem stroke (or pontine infarction) was made. I was left without movement of any kind, including that necessary for speech and, at that stage, for breathing which was aided by a ventilator. Not only was I deprived the comfort of eating, but my nutrition entered my body via drips resulting in painful and tender wrists. I couldn't comprehend the long-term implications. Not being able to move, not being able to eat, not being able to talk – surely there must be some mistake . . .

Apart from the jumble of machinery which distinguished my room from a typical hospital room, there were microphones which operated all night to monitor my heartbeat from a machine which continuously beeped and which graphically displayed my heartbeat in green. I was obviously critically ill but my distress concerned my growing absence from London and how this would affect my chances of getting the job I so wanted and at which I was confident I could do well.

I remember clearly, when coming to my senses in a stifling hot Singapore hospital bed, thinking that those moving about in wheelchairs were the 'lucky' ones, compared to me, motionless in my sweaty hospital bed. I longed for a wheelchair too (how times had changed) and how modest was such an ambition.

But hell! Was it hot there! Even for a man who likes the heat, that hospital was stifling. Yet one evening my teeth were chattering so badly that the racket even woke me. Two frowning doctors were standing at the foot of the bed observing me. It was later discovered I had contracted life-threatening pneumonia. I believed it was just another hurdle in a speedy recovery. Had anyone told me that my progress would be measured in years rather than days, I should have thought them quite mad.

Chapter 7

London

Two-and-a-half weeks after falling ill in Singapore I arrived back in London and was taken directly to the National Hospital for Neurology and Neurosurgery in Queen Square. Carmen returned home. I joined four other patients in the intensive care unit, still unaware of just how sick I really was.

Further investigations revealed an extensive brain-stem lesion and a blocked right internal carotid artery, and by now it had been generally agreed that I had indeed suffered a brain-stem stroke, although an identifiable cause could not be, and has never been, established. The clinical diagnosis of 'locked-in syndrome' had been confirmed.

After six weeks in intensive care my condition had stabilised and I was transferred to the Chandler Ward for men and the merciless clock on the wall. For I had no distractions at all then, save for daily visits from my wife and children. These visits always made me cry – so much work, and for this? And I so desperately wanted to hold them and to be home again with them.

I used to cry, too, whenever I had a bath in a bloody sling arrangement because it brought back to me all the things that I had so recently been able to do. Only dear Nurse Velda (who celebrated her birthday while I was there) seemed to understand.

Somehow the weekdays weren't so bad. There were frequent visits from resident doctors and specialists, for I seemed to be something of a curiosity about the place. But the weekends were interminable. All the doctors would bugger off, leaving the ward a desolate place indeed, and leaving me to my own thoughts and loneliness. Rather than just idly watch the barely perceptible hands on the clock at the end of the wall, I would stare at the window opposite and watch the sun creep its way across the glass.

Any information I had about my condition and my prognosis came from the little snippets Carmen was able to glean. I, the patient, was told nothing. All the usual tests and scans were done but it still wasn't clear to the doctors just why I had suffered a brain-stem stroke. I suspect they all thought I was a boozer and yet I wanted to tell them that I believed the cause of my problem was stress. I would always have chosen to run 20 kilometres than endure 20 minutes of stress and I was sure that no one worked with such intensity or for such long headache-inducing hours.

I was learning my first lesson as a patient: whenever dealing with the medical profession in a hospital environment avoid disappointment and just assume that you will be the last to know anything important about yourself.

Days passed slowly in Chandler. There were visits from Carmen and my girls; my brother Steve taking the time to travel the long distance from his home to see me; long, long sleepless nights; the early morning ritual of the other patients going out to buy a newspaper. How I envied them the simple pleasure of getting out in the fresh morning air to walk.

My mother flew to London not long after the onset of my illness. It took a great effort for her to make the journey and it upset me greatly for her to see me in my state. Seeing my mother had always been a source of such happiness in the past.

Our friends were kindness personified. One weekend our friends the Schneidemans invited the entire family, including my mother, down to their holiday house in Dorset. This went well, except that my mother broke a bone in her foot. She returned to Adelaide not long after, leaving behind a family somewhat more relaxed about what lay ahead in Australia after she described the Julia Farr Centre in glowing terms.

At about the same time, and in the same ward, I apparently had a close call one evening due to congestion in my chest which led to difficulty breathing and severe coughing. I had already had several bouts of pneumonia by this time, and still had a bloody great lump of plastic, called a tracheostomy tube, inserted into my throat to aid my breathing.

I was transferred to the intensive care unit where I languished for about two weeks and where my temperature hovered around 40 degrees Celsius, peaking at over 42 degrees. I remember thinking anything below 40 was great.

The staff in Chandler Ward were wonderful, although one particular nurse, Manny, was inordinately attached to my suction machine – a device to clear the airways and aid breathing – and could always scarcely wait to get his hands on it. It consisted of a length of plastic tubing connected to a compressor at one end and at the other, my tracheostomy tube. He would always apply the thing too vigorously sending me into painful paroxysms of coughing.

The days were often tedious and I relished the little excitements. Douglas, one of the male nurses with a new billiard-ball haircut, was caring for a young man suffering from a drug overdose when suddenly the young man sat up and hurled his whole meal, roast spuds and all, at Dougie, calling him an 'effing bastard' at the same time. Poor Dougie could scarcely believe it and spent hours relating the tale of his misfortune to anyone who would listen.

Some days I was taken for a 'walk' in the square opposite the hospital. First I would be lifted out of my hospital bed by a mechanical lifter, a frightening and somewhat demeaning experience. After all, this did involve exposure of one's bum to the world. I was lowered into a wheelchair and strapped in, a serious business involving an ankle belt, a seat belt, and a strap around both my chest and forehead. This last was to prevent my head from bouncing around or falling forward, but I found it especially restrictive and humiliating.

Suitably bound, a pair of sunnies would be jammed on my head and I would be perfunctorily wheeled out of the hospital, down the steps, and bounced (or so it felt) across the pedestrian crossing to the enclosed garden square opposite. Here I would enjoy, at most, an hour of sunshine before being trundled back inside (now seemingly darker and even more foreboding) to my hospital bed to await nightfall. It all seemed a bit surreal, particularly if I had been hallucinating the night before, but I knew that I just had to hang on and get through this unpleasant bit – just plain stubbornness really – because the alternative was pretty awful. I needed to call on every available ounce of self-discipline I could muster then, just to survive each day – and as it turned out, this daily survival thing went on for years. But I didn't realise what lay ahead. I did however know that there wasn't a magical cure for my ills. So every interminable day I would resume my position as the man clinging to the window ledge of a skyscraper and just tense myself up and hold on. And I got through the horrors a day at a time, believing that in any event I would be one day closer to better times.

A distraction of any kind was most welcome. I was grateful whenever the nurses were kind enough to wash my hair. This meant attention, and could chew up a good 45 minutes or so. Hair washing involved cupping my head in a sort of stainless-steel contraption at the end of my bed, and then applying warm water. Apart from being a pleasant sensation in itself, it distracted me from the distressing sight of my muscle fibre just wasting away bit by bit, every day. My feet were so sensitive by now that I couldn't even bear the weight of the sheets on them, and they had begun to turn inwards. The response was to encase both legs to the knee in plaster to straighten my feet! Needless to say, my sleep patterns and general health suffered from just lying on my back with these great weights on my legs.

I had so few distractions then; no retreating inside my

favourite television programme – because I had no TV – or picking up a treasured book or checking the newspaper because I couldn't, and still can't, read print paper of any kind. They were bloody awful times actually with little let up from the daily horror of it all.

I heard others talk of the hospital swimming pool and in my mind's eye I pictured a beautiful pool surrounded by sloping lush green lawns. I imagined myself swimming gentle laps, up and down, up and down. I also believed at that time that I had a cold room adjoining my own, in which I kept chilled drinks for visiting nephews or my own dear children. Such was the state of my mind.

I never did find out what the swimming pool looked like but it was probably indoors and half full of piss, while the cool room of my imagination turned out not to contain a well-stocked fridge but was instead some kind of sluice room in which the nurses emptied the ward's urine.

Much of my time during these first few months was spent just trying to come to grips with what had changed in my life. During the early days in this hospital, while strapped in a wheelchair, I had fallen asleep with my head resting on my hands. When I woke, my fingers were pushed above the level of the back of my hands, resembling the legs of a dead spider. I looked down at the contorted hands of a paralysed person. It is difficult to describe just how depressed and frightened I felt then. I knew that I was in big trouble and because I couldn't move or talk, this was a battle in which I had few resources on my side. So, if I was to emerge a winner it had to be from using my head correctly, by working smarter not harder. Life is a state of mind. Here then was the ultimate test of that view.

After about seven months of this I had shown virtually no improvement. This is unusual, since most of one's improvement is expected to have occurred by the first six months. Yet I was still alive in spite of the nature of the stroke I had suffered. Of those who do survive such a stroke, locked-in syndrome is invariably chronic. There are rare reports in the medical literature of recovery, most commonly of a minimal or only moderate degree, but slow improvement can take place over a number of years. I remember seeing two manila folders in the ICU in London, both marked in pencil. One related to an elderly lady and simply said: not expected to recover. She died a few days later. The other folder had my name on it and was marked: expected to recover strongly. It's taking its bloody time.

However, having decided that I would be one of those who recovered, Carmen and I decided to return to Adelaide. In South Australia I could be embraced by the warmth of my extended family in the city where we started out all those not-so-long years ago. We had heard of a place called the Julia Farr Centre, which apparently had a sound reputation for rehabilitation, and my mother had confirmed this. The decision being made, we prepared to leave London.

Chapter 8

Adelaide (Again)

Occupying a position in the leafy eastern suburbs of Adelaide, the Julia Farr Centre is a large complex of buildings, commanding, from its upper floors, panoramic views of the ocean and the Adelaide Hills. It was formerly known as the Home for Incurables, a name which can hardly have filled its residents with confidence and faith. Carmen and I had great hopes of the skilled and experienced staff to aid rehabilitation and in fact we had gambled heavily on this roll of the dice.

Carmen had let our house in London and managed to sell our beautiful schooner *Sulara* in the depths of a recession, so at least, for now, we didn't have money worries. Yet once upon a time I had believed that financial concerns were the worst worries a person could have.

I began life in Julia Farr in Room 13, an intensive care room where the nurses viewed you from behind a glass window. I had a splendid view of the Adelaide Hills and of the Waite Agricultural Research Institute and a man on one side who made animal noises and on the other, a chap with an incessant cough and associated rattle. It all made for a fairly uplifting environment.

One night I had been sat outside on the balcony of this multi-storeyed grey brick institution, practising my neck movements – over and over and over – when one of the nurses walked up and pointed out a purple light that was visible in the distance. It was a still, clear night, so we could see for quite a way.

'I think it's Fullarton Road,' she said.

It was a moment of lip-biting loneliness and sadness for me because I knew that road well, had driven along it often, and it brought home to me, again, that there was a whole world of activity going on out there, without me.

Even though I still could not move, walk or speak, I had brought with me from London an alphabet board, and I had adopted the 'eyes up for yes, eyes down for no' system, which meant that I could communicate passably, provided people were willing to use the board. I was at the mercy of their patience and their skill at timing the letters as they were read to me. Some staff could not (or would not) ever use my alphabet board which involves dividing the alphabet into five columns, each headed by a vowel and ascribed a number from one to five. Thus, a, e, i, o, u correspond to the numbers 1, 2, 3, 4, 5. The letters of the alphabet in each column continue until the next vowel is reached, thus the first column consists of the letters a,b,c,d. When someone calls out the numbers 1 to 5, I am able to indicate with eye movement which number (column) I want, and then if the letters in that column are read out, I again signal with my eyes when the desired letter is reached. In this way I am able to spell out a message. With patience and practice I am able to reach a fair speed. When staff refused to use the alphabet board they robbed me of any way of communicating with them. To win a point against a speechless quadriplegic isn't much of a win at all.

Sleeping wasn't so bad by now, although waking each morning to the realisation that this was not all a terrible nightmare was quite awful. One morning I glanced through the charge sheets which were left within my field of vision, and to my horror read the words: we nearly lost him that time. That didn't make sleep any easier for the next few nights, but it did help with the hallucinations, the result of a fevered brain. On waking or in the night I would see things that weren't there. Cruelly in these hallucinations, I was able to walk and talk.

I spent these early weeks, sustained by the inspiring view and visits from my wife and children, my parents, and my brother and his family. I survived my time under close medical surveillance, and was promoted to the other side of the building to Room 8, and a view of the sea in the distance. How I love the sea.

It was after about 12 months back in Adelaide, and therefore some 19 months after my stroke, that a workable speech therapy programme was able to be put in place at Julia Farr, since prior to that all the muscles necessary for articulation were completely paralysed.During those early months in London, my progress had been infinitesimally small. I was as weak as a kitten, with now a completely wasted body. I could only raise a small flicker of movement from my tongue and my right thumb. I deeply resented having a gastrostomy tube for feeding directly into my stomach, and a tracheostomy tube to aid my breathing inserted into my throat. Once in Adelaide, however, my general health improved, and after about 15 months it was possible to have the tracheostomy tube removed. I was then able to embark on a course of hydrotherapy, which had been impossible prior to this because of the danger of infection.I employed a private physiotherapist, Susan Hillier, who was very bright, well qualified and capable. Once more Carmen had investigated the options and chosen just the right person. The hospital's own physiotherapists were perfectly competent but there were just too few of them. Susan visited me twice weekly, and I had hydrotherapy once weekly. Hydrotherapy was marvellous for many reasons, but principally because it made me feel alive again.

I still did not know how long my rehabilitation would take, nor how long I would remain a resident of the Julia Farr Centre. There were many capable and caring staff at Julia Farr who warrant praise, just as a few deserve vilification. The overwhelming challenge seemed to be one of staff shortages.

My days in Julia Farr would usually start at about 3 am with the excruciating pain of flesh on flesh. This would result from one limb partially crossing another during the night and, being paralysed, there was nothing I could do about it. (Next time you see a person in a wheelchair, do not assume, as I have done in the past, that he or she feels no pain. If they are anything like me, they will be feeling everything, in spite of their paralysis.) So I lay in the early morning gloom, filling in the hours by watching the dawn slowly light up the curtains in my room, waiting for the mobilisation that brought relief from my pain, which usually came with the final night-shift round at 6 am. The night staff had started work at 10.30 pm and during the night each patient would be turned at least twice; once at around 12.30 am and again at about 6 am. If my luck was in, David would be on duty and he would expect me to listen and respond intelligently to his queries about the stock market. I cherished his kindness and respect in a place often too busy to dispense hope.

The early day shift arrived at about 6.30 am and handover from night shift would follow. This tended to be brief in the mornings – about 15 minutes or so – and the staff would then move to shower or bathe residents; everyone, everyday. The moment the nurses started showering, they would turn on the infernal radio. From about 7.15 am, Today's Easy-Listening 5AD blasted out from the bathroom. However, once in the shower I would get my revenge by squirting the nurses with the hand-held shower hose which, apart from providing me with amusement, also allowed me to practise movements in the flat shower-bath which helped to inform me of my progress. Bathed and dressed I was placed in a wheelchair, that most awful of machines, in which I spent all the daytime hours. I loathed it and everything it represented – it was anathema to me, representing my loss of independent mobility. No longer did I envy those in their wheelchairs as I had in Singapore in the early days of my illness. Once in my wheelchair I would go straight onto the computer, either to write some more for this book or to write some letters. Without the computer I think I should have gone mad. It provided me with a diversion from the horror.

And so the rituals of each day passed into afternoon and the arrival of the late shift. The afternoon hand-over was usually a giggly and raucous affair, lasting some 45 minutes. God only knows what they found to talk and laugh about.

The late-shift staff would often put me to bed at about 7 pm, in time for the evening news on the ABC which thankfully was free of bloody advertisements. At other times I would stay working at the computer until as late as 9.30 pm, burying myself in my writing for as long as possible and thus minimising the length of time I would be in bed with no distractions from the awful reality of my condition.

On our return to Adelaide, Carmen had bought a house quite close to the centre, and about twice a week I went 'home'. My visits home usually occurred in the afternoons on Thursdays and late Sunday mornings. These visits were very precious, providing me with the opportunity to see Carmen and the children, and of maintaining the feeling of being connected to my home base, to the world outside the Centre, and to life. The only problem in leaving the hospital was that an Access cab had to be arranged, a modified taxi which caters for wheelchairs. The strapping in which needed to take place – and there was plenty of it – left me in no doubt as to the depths I had fallen.

I was so desperate to get out of the institution that I would manufacture other day trips. First I had to persuade one of the nurses to book me a taxi. One day I concocted the idea of travelling, unattended, into a city-based sports store for a look around and a spot of shopping, although in reality I had no earthly idea what I would buy or how I would manage to transact the purchase once I got there. Unfortunately the taxi driver was suspicious of my little scheme and before we arrived at our destination he had called back to his base for clarification and promptly returned me to my room. I was eventually put on the banned list for cab bookings unless I was going home for a visit or meeting someone.

Then I began to make progress a little faster, albeit still at a snail's pace. Probably the hardest thing for me to do was to open my mouth wide on command, rather than involuntarily. The next most difficult thing was to stick out my tongue, even if only a little bit. Both of these controlled movements, simple for most people and almost impossible for me, are essential for speech. In order to learn to eat and drink again, I had to relearn the far-from-easy task of swallowing. In the meantime, I continued to be sustained by a gastrostomy.

In case you think that I have a set of super-bowels and could last nigh on two years without once calling on the good graces of the nurses, well, no. Sadly, the truth was that every two or three days, usually at my discretion, I would be given two Enemax to get things going, wheeled away on a dunny seat on wheels, and be told to get on with it.

These tedious but life-sustaining daily rituals went on for six long years.

Chapter 9

Reflections on Being a Patient

As a resident of a number of hospitals for several years, and the recipient of the ministrations of countless nurses and other hospital staff, I have been struck by how very sensitive and caring some can be, and how insensitive and thoughtless are others. I was totally reliant on nursing staff for daily care and the quality of such care became crucial to my basic comfort and wellbeing.

Yet there are those with a gravel voice and personality to match who demand a 'yes' or 'no' answer instantly and seem unable to appreciate that even a computer needs time to warm up. Some seem to have the unerring capacity to be unhelpful. Try to imagine how I felt, when I had done a day's laborious writing on the computer, only to have a nurse unknowingly switch the machine off before I had the chance to save my work, thereby losing the lot.

I remember one particular evening when I was about to be turned at midnight by the evening 'raiding party' headed by a nurse whom I couldn't stand. Indeed, I would bristle at the sight of the woman. Unfortunately, I had awoken with a giant (for me) erection hopelessly trapped inside the plastic bottle I had been given for the night. When I was turned pressure was taken off the bottle which acted as though it had just been released from a spring-loaded trap. It somersaulted through the air and the base of the bottle hit me square in the middle of the forehead. Even 'Mrs Hitler' thought that was funny and had to leave the room to disguise her mirth, or so I was later told. I was so convulsed with laughter that I didn't notice her absence. Humour helped keep me sane.

I saw striking examples of the Peter Principle, where the best and most capable hands-on nurses were moved into administrative positions for which they may not have been suited, and others who, although they must at some time or other have been through nursing training, seemed to be totally bereft of nursing skills.

Many times I was in an impossibly uncomfortable position when a nurse entered my room, dispensed medication – often to me – and then walked straight out again, leaving me to my discomfort for hours. Or I might have had, say, both feet hanging out of the bed so that a nurse collided with them and yet still didn't notice. It was a peculiarly vulnerable feeling to come back from swimming in wet togs and to be parked by the cab driver in my room for a couple of hours and left to stare at a blank wall. Although I could hear people moving along the corridor I was completely powerless either verbally or physically to get their attention and improve my circumstances.

I was generally placed in a room directly opposite a nurses' station supposedly to prevent me from choking, or worse. Yet I swear I could have died a dozen times or more before my imminent demise would be heard above the chatter.

The best nurses were those who remembered the details of patients' needs, who remembered I always wore glasses to watch television; who could be caring without being patronising. I resented being fondled too much while they muttered 'there, there'. But it was delightful to have a nurse who could offer an intelligent comment. In the early years of my illness a nurse named Carina was wonderful to me. Whether it was the share prices I wanted read, help with an exercise programme, or a wheelchair tyre needing more air, Carina would be there to help. Sadly she moved to another hospital.

I missed her dedicated care. Generally the nursing staff, especially those on night shift, were a friendly, good-natured lot with whom I shared a laugh.

Yet I sometimes wonder just how many of the nurses understood what being a quadriplegic – and one without speech – really meant. All the pushing, shoving and yanking would seem to suggest otherwise. Some of the practices I have described above could be dismissed as simply careless or thoughtless, (and I appreciate that all nursing staff at times are overworked and stressed). Nevertheless there are some staff whose single-minded heedlessness amounted at best to neglect, and at worst to a terrible abuse of power.

Chapter 10

The Fight Begins

Every day, I still had to rely on the kindness, goodwill and vigilance of others in order to survive. But I had a revelation, and it came to me by degrees. It wasn't so much the things I couldn't do that were important, but rather, if I was going to get out of the mess, I had to concentrate on the things I could do. I had to concentrate on my strengths, not my weaknesses, for I would surely perish if I panicked and floundered about. Some four or five years elapsed before I realised that this was now the way I must approach things. In short, if life is a state of mind then this must be the state of mind for me.

To say that I wanted to get out of that institution would be a vast understatement. In fact I lay awake at night imagining the day I would finally drive out through the gates forever. Just as each hospital inmate had a carefully planned medication regime, so each should have had a meticulously planned (and agreed) exit strategy. I feel very strongly about this. If patients had a goal to strive toward it would prevent much of the aimless existing which occurs in places such as the one in which I found myself, and from which I was forced after six or more long years to conduct my own exit strategy. Incidentally, the cost saving to the community of moving people from a taxpayer-funded hospital, and into some form of tax-paying employment within the community, would be huge.

I continued writing with the aid of a computer, by means of a single switch which I operated with the index finger of my right hand. Once in my wheelchair I could be pushed up to the computer for a day's typing, broken only by spells of physio. My computer allowed me to communicate with staff, and to write letters to my family, albeit very slowly – three to four days writing one letter was fairly commonplace.

Much has been written about just how long after a stroke one can expect significant recovery to occur. I was rapidly learning the value of persistence and repetition, and that if my brain could not command my muscles to generate a desired movement, then repetition eventually would. Very simply this involved going over and over and over a particular exercise in the hope that other muscle groups would join in. I took absolutely every opportunity to exercise. Exercise, however minimal, was surely better than just vegetating. So, in the half light before I was taken off for a bath in the morning, I would sometimes do as many as 1500 repetitions of a shrug-like movement of my right shoulder. On my way home in a taxi after an outing, there would be certain spots on the road where I would work to elevate my leg. To gain head control, I would move my head from side to side, while maintaining my head in an upright position. For years I could do only 100 a day, but one amazing day I completed 450. So 500 then became the benchmark. In the portable bath each morning I would try to raise my right hand to a point on my chest above my plastic gastrostomy button and back down on to the bath again, without touching my side. Using my elbow as a fulcrum I could j-u-s-t do this, and would continue until the muscles were completely fatigued – usually as few as half a dozen would exhaust me.

Persistence is a quality I had always valued. When I was a young beltman with the Portsea SLSC in February 1972, there was a dangerous surf running and a young man had managed to get himself into danger when a sandbar gave way. He was stranded about 200 metres from shore in white water, which meant not only that the line I was towing out to him had a huge bow in it from the strong side current, but also that the bubbles were a good six inches above the level of the water's surface. As I swam out I planned to approach him with caution because he was already in a state of panic. I stood about ten metres away to catch my breath and also to avoid him throwing his arms around me and dragging us both down. I introduced myself and told him what I was about. He calmed down, allowing me to grab him from behind and signal to shore that we were ready to be towed back. However the rope must have caught under a rock because no sooner did the lifesavers start pulling us toward shore than we were pulled straight under, necessitating my pulling the pin on the harness that I was wearing and casting us both adrift in the swirling water.

This is where persistence came in, for I had resolved that I would save this bloke, that he could be talked around eventually. Well, eventually was the operative word because it was the best part of an hour in that swirling water before another line could be sent from shore. But by sticking to my plan, and talking calmly and reasonably, we eventually made it to shore. Persistence had saved that young swimmer. And it would save me now, too.

My physical skills seemed to improve after repetitive

exercise. I imagined my limb as a rusty gate – the more it was moved the easier it became, and if one applied a little oil (regenerating nerves) then maybe it would work almost as it once had.

In early 1997 I had built for me a standing frame which went a long way toward preventing the onset of osteoporosis, but didn't do much else. The aim was to use it for at least half an hour at a time, every day. The difficulties in doing so were considerable, not least of which was simply trying to organise the two staff necessary to put me on and take me off it. It was also very tiring, exhausting in fact, particularly at first. I found there was a world of difference between sitting in a chair or lying in bed and standing on the frame. I likened this experience to trying to pick up a piece of over-ripe fruit by the stem and hoping that it (muscles, ligaments, bones) all held together without tearing or breaking.

Indeed, the first few times I blacked out and came within an ace of vomiting. With saliva streaming from my mouth, I would be lumbered back to my room and a pulse taken (sometimes with great difficulty) from my cold and sweaty wrist. But in time this corrected itself. For some years after my stroke my right leg was significantly shorter than the left, which made standing in the frame very painful.

Then in late 1997 I transferred to a more dynamic form of

standing frame, the Pixel. This machine allowed the exercising of arms, legs, buttocks and stomach while being elevated into a standing position, and vital neck and torso exercises and legs, in particular, once upright.

I would strongly recommend anyone in my position to buy their own Likon machine which electronically stimulates muscle causing it to contract. I have tried many different therapies but only two things, oxygen drops and the Likon machine, have consistently worked for me.

I think the major advantage of the machine is that it allows muscles to be built up to a point from which the body can take over. I believe that muscles allowed to just idle will simply atrophy. The Likon allows separate muscles to be exercised thoroughly, albeit the muscle contractions are electronically stimulated. Long after the body is fatigued from exertion, the Likon can be used selectively on individual muscle groupings. The machine itself is completely portable and can be used anywhere, any time, on just about any muscle group; pretty important advantages really. It liberated me, allowing me to feel that I was in control of at least a few movements which, after so many years of inactivity, made it worthwhile in itself. And, after exercise, hydrotherapy. Tired and aching limbs and joints can be moved about so much easier in the supportive water, especially if it is warm.

My exercise regime at Julia Farr involved 90-minute physiotherapy sessions, four or more times a week, to stretch my muscles; standing on the purpose-built frame for up to an hour at a time three or more times a week to strengthen my muscles and bones; using the Likon machine whenever possible to a maximum of three hours a day; and, every Sunday morning, hydrotherapy with my dear brother Steve and his wife Stephanie. I had fought for additional hydrotherapy and while this was therapeutic, it just wasn't for long enough given that the rest of the time I sat around with leaden limbs. And I grew sick of the amount of time it took each and every week to convince others to bend the rules sufficiently to enable me to go to hydrotherapy twice each week. The conventional wisdom for a pontine stroke victim is that there's no hope of improvement so don't rock the boat. This sort of direct opposition occurred whenever I attempted to try and secure additional services to aid my recovery. In short, I was not only battling my own body, whose natural tendency it was to take the line of least resistance and do nothing, but I was also battling entrenched attitudes and work practices.

While my weekly regime may seem like a lot of exercise, remember that there were long periods of complete inactivity in between, when I just sat. All of this therapy only made sense if I believed in what I was doing, if I was confident that I would improve.

I also tried an exercise bike, upon which a gentleman from Technical Aid for the Disabled had spent many hours building a frame with lots of straps to support me while someone moved my feet on the pedals. I had great hopes for this machine but it just hurt my bum too much to sit on the bike and it was too ungainly for frequent use. It was eventually consigned to the room for white elephants.

Then I became wildly enthusiastic about oxygen. I had been frequently admitted to the Royal Adelaide Hospital for severe chest infections. There they had a hyperbaric chamber which delivered oxygen under pressure, much like a marine decompression chamber, and while in the RAH intensive care unit I had been continuously receiving six litres of oxygen an hour. For the first time since my stroke, I received an exogenous boost to my performance without having to precede it with a great deal of graft and hard work. On my return from the RAH following my initial visit I could, for example, touch the tip of each finger on my left (and least mobile) hand with the tip of my thumb. Impressive indeed. I became fervent about this, particularly when a lovely young nurse named Jane lent me some reading matter which indicated pure oxygen, or rather heavy doses of oxygen, had brought similar results in the US. But it was to no avail. The RAH rejected the findings in the US because they felt the research was not rigorous. No amount of letters, phone calls or appointments changed this. I was deeply disappointed for I believed it meant starting again, right from square one.

Instead I used liquified oxygen drops in my flush water after every feed, and took Barley Green, an internal flush supplement, once a day, again thanks to Jane and her friend Bronwyn. The theory is relatively simple: bugs don't survive in an oxygenated environment. I continue to use the oxygen drops to this day. The oxygen drops help me to stay well and the Likon machine allows me to exercise.

Finally, the Triflo. This is a small device designed to improve and to measure the capacity of the lungs, and consists primarily of a tube through which one can inhale and exhale, and three lightweight balls (about one quarter the size of table-tennis balls) which move up through three lightweight plastic tubes as one inhales. This can be more effectively accomplished when standing. Following my stroke, I took very shallow breaths due to my limited lung capacity, which was only going to get worse the longer I remained in a wheelchair. I remember an attractive young medical student suggesting I use the Triflo one day. As she moved away to attend to another matter she mumbled to Ian, a paramedical aide, that he should let me inhale and then see if the balls moved. Quick as a flash, he donned a rubber glove and squatted down in front of the frame with his right hand held in a sort of cupping motion and said,

'Ready'. The girl whirled around and asked him what he was doing. He innocently replied that he was waiting for her to get me to inhale 'to see if my balls moved'. I laughed so hard I nearly fell out of the frame.

About four or five years after my stroke I was invited by Susan Hillier, my physiotherapist, to present a paper to a group of Feldon Kris physiotherapists. I wrote of what I had learned, of my experience as a locked-in patient and what might help others in a similar situation. I wrote of the oxygen drops that I took twice a day with my feed; that kept me well and allowed me to increase my exercise programme. Before oxygen drops, at the onset of a cold or chest infection, I eased up the exercises for a day or so and immediately started a course of antibiotics, which would fix the infection but do precious little for my body's ability to produce antibodies and thus fight the infection itself.

At the time of writing the presentation I had been diagnosed by the local physician as having yet another bloody chest infection. On waking, I registered an oxygen saturation level in the high 70s instead of within the normal range in the high 90s. I had a colleague's wedding to attend in London a few weeks later, and I knew that the airlines wouldn't take me if I had a chest infection. So I tested my faith in oxygen drops and declined the antibiotics offered.

Within two days my chest had cleared and my oxygen levels had climbed back up to the mid 90s on the oximeter, and I was more convinced than ever of the effectiveness of oxygen drops.

I knew the physiotherapy fraternity was far from convinced of the efficacy of electrical-stimulation massage but I told them that the Likon machine had consistently worked for me and that the pedal machine was also excellent. It doesn't aim to build up muscles but aids blood circulation to combat the hideous bone-seeping cold that envelops a motionless person.

I spent hours and hours lying idly on my bed in the institution listening to tapes by Zig Ziglar, an American motivational speaker. Over and over I would listen to them, especially on Sunday. I think everyone else thought I was a little crazy but I found his philosophy valuable and inspiring. Zig Ziglar said that it is your attitude not your aptitude which determines your ultimate altitude. He helped me stay positive which was vital and not all that difficult given that I really believed in a favourable outcome. The choice confronting me was a stark one. I could effectively throw away my life, the one thing that really belonged to me, by staying where I was, away from my home and my family. I would continue my complete dependence on other people, who were sometimes not well disposed toward assisting me, and subscribe to the conventional wisdom that people in my position were scrap-heap material – knackered, finished. *Or* I could strive with every available muscle and nerve fibre for a better outcome.

Repeatedly, Zig Ziglar's message was drilled home: I must identify my goals, and my present status. This would clarify what steps were necessary to reach my goal; in my case, to walk. Other key messages of the tapes were self belief and avoidance of procrastination or detours: once the goal was identified, then simply work toward it – no mucking about. The concept of 'cannot' does not exist.

In my case, the very first step was to improve my self-image, and I did this in two ways. Firstly, and most importantly, I resolved to throw away all my tracksuits. The institution encouraged their use (presumably because they were easy for the nurses to slip on and off), but they did absolutely nothing for my self-image. If I was to have a chance of coming up with solutions and ideas, then I must create the right environment, conducive to such thoughts. Slopping around in a tracksuit identified me as a patient, a man in exile, separated from the world outside. So I insisted on wearing normal clothes every day, even on those days when I knew I would be working at my computer all day and have no visitors.

The other important stand that I took to restore my sense of self was to cease all medication except vitamins but including the mind-numbing relaxant drugs. I faced great opposition, particularly from the nursing staff, who would obviously prefer to care for a person in a relaxed (did I hear the word 'vegetative' mentioned?) state, than a person who is lively and challenging.

Clonazepam is a muscle-relaxant drug originally prescribed to dampen down the involuntary movement in my left eye. Other potential remedies had been attempted: pulling the top eyelid down and stitching it to the cheek below, and when that failed, sticking a needle into my eye and filling the ocular cavity with a botulism mix known as Botox, designed to paralyse the muscles causing the jumping. Both these procedures were painful and neither successful; I still have a wildly jumping eye.

Regrettably the clonazepam wasn't discerning and every other muscle was relaxed as well. Fortunately we had a physiotherapist by the name of Gael Harrison attached to our section who opposed the conventional wisdom and told me that I would never walk while taking clonazepam. That decided me and I set about weaning myself. That brought 'normality' another step closer for me. Normal clothes and no drugs – I wasn't ready for the scrap heap just yet.

However, I was then plagued by fears of all kinds – that

things would never be the same again, that I had risked too much. I had periods of feeling down, especially late at night, when my fledgling sense of self esteem seemed fragile. But at other times I knew that by making these two changes I retained some autonomy over my life, and that I must keep my nerve. A lot would depend on what I did from here.

There didn't seem to be any plan for my discharge from Julia Farr. Rather, there was a casual acceptance of the status quo – that is, I had drawn a bummer card and there wasn't much that could be done about it.

Gradually, I began to venture more frequently outside the four walls of the institution. I also began to socialise more, mostly in the company of one of the nurses, my dear friend Maureen, blessed with a wonderful sense of humour and a huge heart. She accompanied me as I played cards with my mates, took day trips, and went out for meals where I watched my friends eat and listened to their chatter.

This was a very big step, for it forced me to meet people that I hadn't met in years and to face them as silent and motionless as a statue. Seeing their response heightened my sense of loss. What is more, I had to view them, and indeed the whole world, from a sitting position. I didn't like it all that much, nor did I like having to depend on others for absolutely every damn thing. Having to be pushed everywhere was annoying, but then on meeting someone, I was unable to speak or move other than to leer at them and, as I once heard it put, to display about as much co-ordination as a dislocated elbow. This was even more distressing.

I remember two situations particularly clearly. We were taken to hydrotherapy aboard one of those large buses that are occasionally seen trundling around chock-full of unfortunate-looking people. And then it hit me. *I* was one of those staring out of the bus at the world of the normal. Sometimes I felt as if my heart would break.

Also, I dribbled all the time, as in *all* the time. I had been pushed down to the local shops one afternoon and parked outside while my carer bought himself an ice cream. I waited, unable to swallow, and the overflow of saliva flooded from my mouth. Unfortunately this poor little fellow walked out of the shop to be greeted not only by the sight of a cripple in a wheelchair, but a furiously dribbling cripple. He looked at me horrified and backed away and I wondered if I had scarred him for life. It was such an absurd situation and I responded in one of the only ways I could; I burst into uncontrollable laughter.

Getting out and doing more 'normal' things gradually became easier and with my tracksuit discarded and a drug-free brain I was ready for my next step. It seemed to all come down to the value of five minutes: the difference between watching the clock wishing each day away, or wishing time would slow because there is so much to do. I had rediscovered a sense of urgency, of *impatience*, that seemed crucial to building a new and exciting life. I could no longer tolerate the bland, featureless existence that came with slippers and daytime TV.

I prepared to escape.

Chapter 11

Early Days away from JF

My life had been scythed in two. I could not repair the damage but I refused to accept my productive life was over. I was desperate to break out and do something with this other half of my life.

If I was going to escape, then it was essential that I didn't have anyone holding me back 'for my own good', so absolute secrecy was maintained, and I didn't even tell my family or the therapists. I believed therapies were more concerned with improving the functionality of my existing capabilities than encouraging new skills and, in addition, many of the therapists were obstructive.

What I did was choose an ally and confidante, my nurse and friend Maureen, and we worked together to obtain suitable accommodation for me in the real world. In the grim early days of institutional life, Maureen always seemed nearby. Now she facilitated my departure. My visual impairment meant I couldn't read the classified section of the newspaper and I couldn't, of course, make the necessary phone calls for appointments. Instead I escaped from the institution to visit the few rental selections I had made via an Access cab assisted by the drivers who colluded (unknowingly) by pushing me around. This little exercise was another small step toward restoring my vitality as an individual. I had always loved the sea and eventually I decided on a flat on the sea-front, the perfect change from the monotony and drabness of the institution. Having found a place to live, Maureen and I then had to adapt it to meet my needs. This proved to be a time consuming and hideously expensive thing to do. It needed to cater for everyday living for the carers as well as myself. And I needed a hospital environment replicated to meet any potential emergency.

I had a special steel gantry and lifting device built, designed to help me walk again. Not only was there nothing even remotely like this in the institution where I had lived, but I often chuckled to myself at the sheer impossibility of negotiating such vital equipment through the labyrinthine corridors of bureaucracy. To this day I still have a framed 'defective' sticker hanging on the wall in the room where the gantry is situated. This was stuck on a standing frame which had been built for me at my expense, but which the Julia Farr physiotherapist decided was unsafe and it was confiscated. I think I re-defined frustration at Julia Farr.

In case you're wondering why I just didn't go home, it is because my wife Carmen had decided to live 800 kilometres away in Melbourne and so the family house was tidied up and sold. And no, I didn't even see it coming. Therefore I was without my wife and children and without a home to escape to. I was thrown back on to the property market to do things I hadn't done for over a quarter of a century. In a weak moment, half dazed with illness, I had signed over my Power of Attorney to Carmen. Now I wanted it back. All my plans for the future depended on this. Fortunately Carmen had no objections and I convinced a lawyer, a dapper chap in a dark-blue pin-striped suit, that I was legally sane. I immediately opened a cheque account and experienced the delight of once again controlling my money.

I had found a residence, a flat in West Lakes near the sea, but finding appropriate carers was arguably the biggest challenge to overcome. At times I found myself frozen into inaction by vague half-thought-through fears that it would be impossible to survive away from the hospital. Who would be there when I needed help? No one was questioning the need for 24-hour care. Perhaps I'd be better off in an institution where that was provided with minimal input from me.

Balls! Of course it could be done. I must leave the place in which I felt a captive in every sense. I had to maintain my dignity, or what there was left of it, and stay true to myself, because if I allowed myself to become one of the tracksuit-and-slipper brigade then I was surely lost for good.

Eventually the big day dawned, and after a final shower from my favourite nurse Nick, I savoured the moment and farewelled my life at Julia Farr. However it was not a clean break. For the first weeks of my new-found freedom I spent from Friday morning to Monday night at my new home with my carer(s) but for the rest of the week I remained at the institution. I had little appetite for this form of phased withdrawal but I realised safety was a priority and keeping a bet on each side seemed logical if unpalatable.

So impatient had I been to leave that in early 1998 I checked myself out from the institution without the necessary carer arrangements in place. This meant that initially I relied heavily on the good graces and kindness of my guardian angel, Maureen. She was assisted by her friend Dorothy, who I grew to like very much. I have the most enormous gratitude for the assistance Maureen offered over a long time, but especially during this period of great change.

I had found a home away from institutional restrictions and now I set about finding a suitable property in which I could establish a small business and thus allow my carers the day-time hours to pursue their own interests, and allow me to make my day-time carer (my secretary) tax-effective. So every time my head fell down, or I coughed myself out of position, the care was tax-deductible.

I rented three rooms of an old house with a good business address: one room for me, one for the secretaries, and one for housing my exercise equipment, photographs, wine, and other memorabilia. At first I envisaged running a simple consultancy for small businesses whereby people would come to me with their business problems, I would listen, and then type up a report on the computer for them. All of this I could do, but I lived in Adelaide, not New York, and no rush of clients was forthcoming. So, by degrees, I developed into a writer and publisher of a business newsletter, *Hermes*. This was something I could do, for it essentially involved knowledge, experience and time to think (something I had in abundance) and then tap-tap-tapping out information and advice using my index finger and a computer. I had two efficient secretaries who transformed what I had written into a professional-looking newsletter which was sent to businesses which had subscribed.

Having an office large enough to house equipment allowed me to exercise whenever I wanted. For years my exercise had been restricted to small doses at designated times and I had been distressed by the knowledge that my opportunities to retain or improve my physical skills had been limited. In my own premises I could exercise at will.

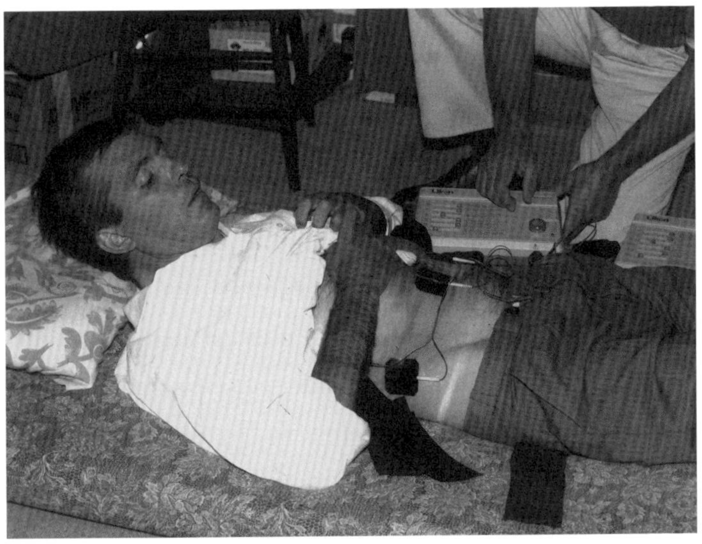

Exercise session with Ian using the Likon machine to exercise abdominal muscles, at the office, Adelaide, 1999

I placed newspaper advertisements for carers and elicited a huge response. From the many interviews one applicant stood out, an Irish lad named Steve who for immigration reasons could only stay for three months. He was small in stature and jocular and worked 16 hours a day caring for me.

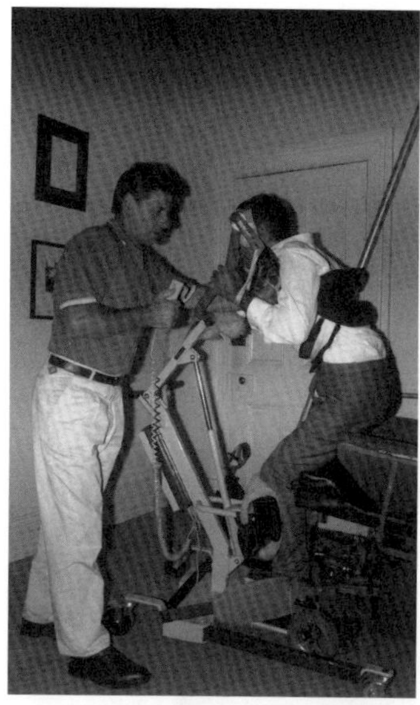
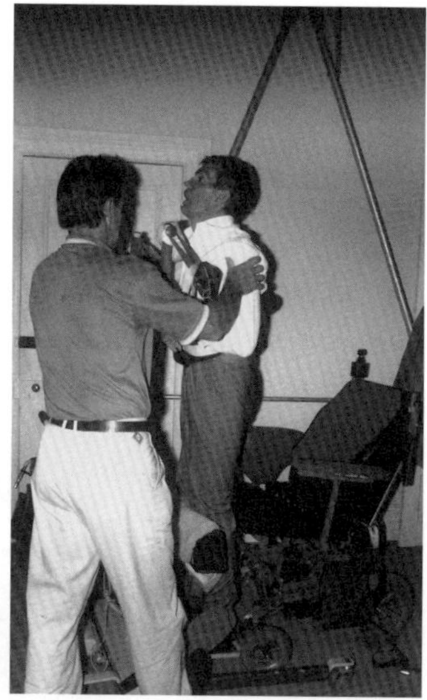

Ian assists me into an upright position using the standing frame, at the office, Adelaide, 1999

Those few months in my own flat with Steve to care for me were blissful. Now I could decide when to go to bed and when to rise, and most importantly I returned to my new home from the office each night to my own bed rather than a hospital bed. These may seem insignificant changes but they were hugely important to me following years of sleeping each night in a bed that wasn't my own, having every moment constrained, regimented and organised. I discovered that at night I needed a carer much less than I had imagined. There were many nights when I didn't call my carer to change my bottle or relieve pressure on a limb, and

I enjoyed more restful evenings in my own bed than I ever did in a hospital environment where, for example, all patients had been routinely turned at midnight whether they needed it or not.

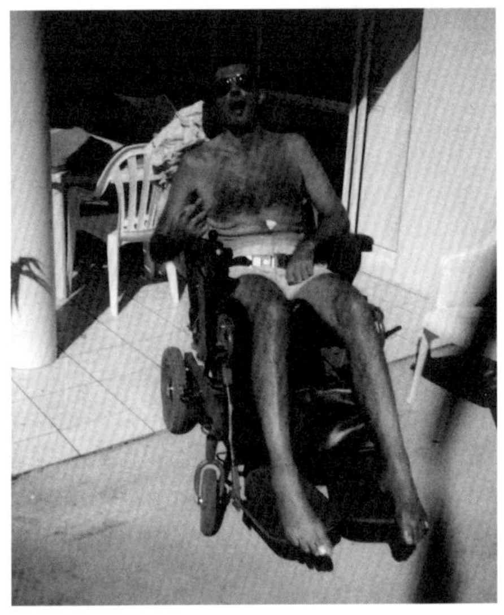

Enjoying the sun on holiday, Queensland, 2000

And I had fun. I recall one day sitting inside with Steve while a neighbour exercised on the lawn outside my window. I indicated to Steve that my crutch area was tight and needed adjusting. I waited until the neighbour was watching and Steve had his hand far down my trousers. I then gripped his hand between my arm and my body, thus preventing him from extracting it, and for the neighbour's benefit I feigned a look of ecstatic enjoyment. The poor chap reacted as though I had put an electric current up his arm. I guess from the neighbour's viewpoint this must have looked odd indeed. I was so creased up with laughter I no longer noticed him.

While I was living by the sea at West Lakes I would go swimming with Ian, an exercise-therapist who also responded to my advertisements for carers. Ian was employed to organise my exercise regime but soon revealed skills in other areas. He advised me about nutrition and increased my mobility by modifying a normal plastic shower chair by fitting strong detachable axles to which wheelbarrow wheels were added for negotiating the sand. I remember in

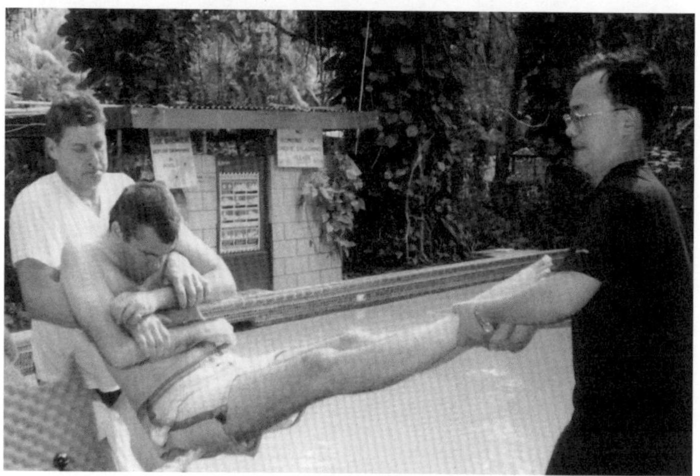

About to be taken for a swim while on holiday, Airlie Beach, Queensland, 2000

particular a perfect summer's day as Ian took me out in my chair, pushing me along the firm sand near the water's edge in the beautiful sunshine as I sucked in great lungfuls of salt-laden air. Although risky because of the danger of inhaling water I was taken swimming in the sea wearing a life jacket. This necessitated considerable preparation and relied on Ian's great strength. He seemed to understand not only my need to exercise but my need to push the limits. The chair also made beach holidays possible because once I had the chair stowed as luggage I could go anywhere. This was not life in an institution; this was why I had fought to escape.

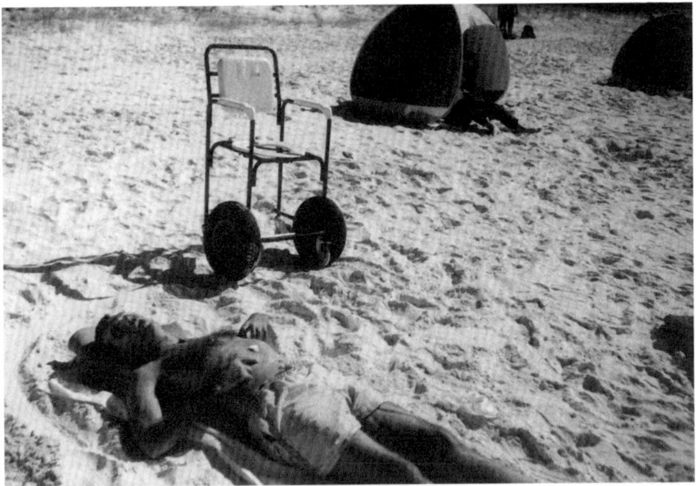

On holiday in Queensland, 2000. Note the shower chair with wheelbarrow wheels used to negotiate the sand and enter the water

I had first met Simona 'Sam' Angeletti when I worked in Sydney 20 years earlier and had developed strong feelings towards her. But she was recently married and by then I had a family of my own and felt my responsibilities very keenly – especially to my children for whom setting a good example was of great importance to me. Over the long years in Julia Farr, I had been thinking of Simona, thinking I wanted to see her. I knew she had separated from her husband before I left for London in 1983 but I didn't know where she lived and it was likely that if I did manage to find her she would now be married and have a family. But it was *possible* that Simona was still single, and so on the principle of 'nothing ventured nothing gained' I set about trying to find her. I laboured for a while under the incorrect spelling of her surname but once my brain had straightened out this little problem, progress was quite swift.

Aided by Ian (who, not for the first time, was my 'legs' in this endeavour), I reasoned that the last time I had spoken with Simona nearly 20 years before, she had been of voting age and so, presumably, had her husband. I then obtained a map of the city in which she had lived all those years ago. Even though I couldn't remember exactly where she lived, I narrowed the search by telling Ian in which electoral areas she didn't live! Once found, it was a simple step to identify the husband's name (because he would have been at the same address) and then a check of the most recent electoral roll would more than likely reveal where he now lived. This turned out to be so.

Regrettably he had a silent phone number so something as simple as recourse to a telephone was entirely useless. So finally, of necessity, I used the address on the electoral roll and wrote to Simona's ex-husband explaining my circumstances. Fortunately he was a decent man and passed the message on to Simona that I was looking for her. I remember the day she rang from her home in Rome. Ian was giving me some exercises at the time and he said quietly in my ear 'Is that who I think it is?'

It is difficult to overstate the difference Simona has made to my life. She has turned my life around and given me the confidence to lead a more or less normal existence. On top of that she has such wonderful values and I love her for that, and I am so very proud of her. I think the most important single thing is that she always, but always, puts me first! I very much believe in 'quid pro quo' – give as you get – and I hope I repay in full the love and kindness Simona has shown me.

Try to imagine what life was like for me before Simona. Unable to walk, talk or eat, I basically worked and slept – in short, I lived for my work. I had literally nothing better to

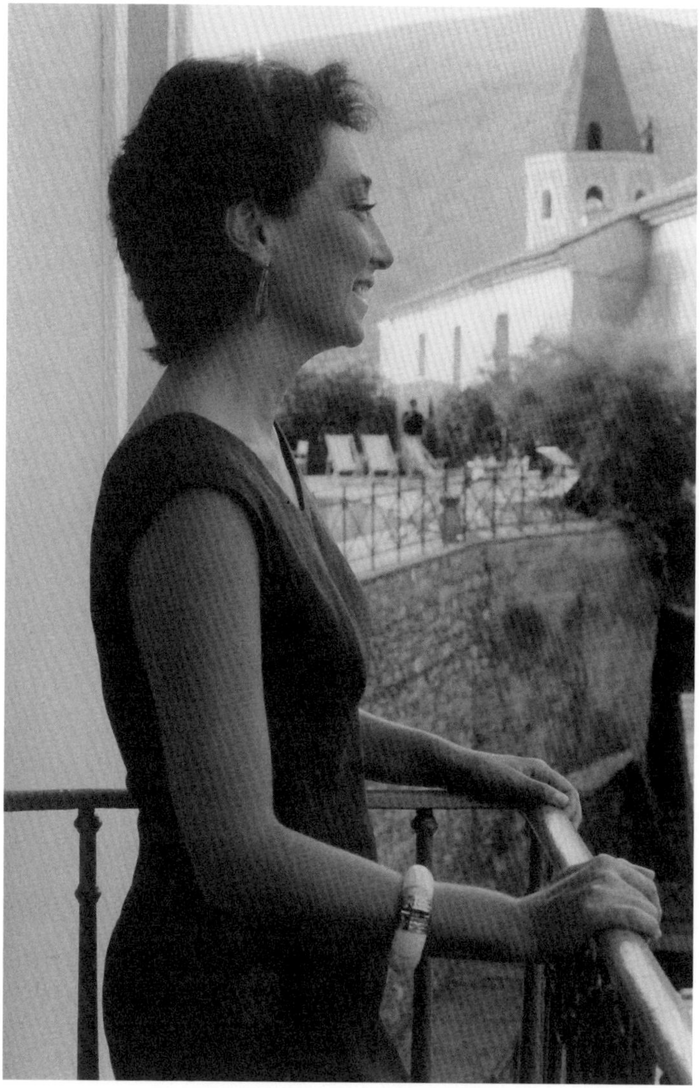

My darling Simona, Italy, 1996

do, seven days a week. Apart from being in love with her anyway (more than anyone on the planet if truth be known) she returned structure and dignity to my life.

I didn't like my environment so I changed it. I checked myself out of hospital, rented my own flat, hired my own carers, started my own business, and I found Simona. I had rejoined the human race.

Chapter 12

Simona's story

It was a winter's day in 1980; I was 21 and newly and happily married. Life was good and the future looked bright. I loved my job and my friends. But life is unpredictable, and sometimes things happen when you least expect them, events that make you question your life choices. Little did I know that from that day my life was to take a different turn; that I would meet someone who would dictate my destiny.

I was an accounts clerk for Meares & Philips, a stock broking firm in the beautiful city of Sydney. I was developing professionally under the guidance of the partners. I knew my place. In those days there was no calling your bosses by their first name, no wearing jeans to work. The offices were carpeted, hushed and staid. On this normal day in an office world I remember approaching the partners to get some cheques signed and to my astonishment saw the most beautiful, gorgeous man I had ever seen sitting on the side of a desk behind one of the partners.

A light brown suit, spectacles and very long legs. My heart stopped and our eyes met for just a moment and I knew I was in trouble. I have never again felt that bite in my heart. Very few people have the ability to bring so much with them, but Peter did. He had it all: intelligence, a sense of humour, good looks, happiness, and youth. He felt positive about life and sparked with energy. He was a knock out. All the girls were in love with him, you could tell. We all melted under one of his smiles or a lifting of those eyebrows. That day, Peter stole my heart and he never gave it back.

In 1983 our lives took different paths for different reasons. My marriage had come to an end and I was about to move to Rome. Leaving Sydney, and Meares & Philips, was devastating. Peter was about to move to London with his family.

It was Sunday 18 February 2001 when a call from Sydney changed my life again. My former husband phoned informing me that a person from Adelaide (a colleague from Meares & Philips) was looking for me. I knew it was Peter. Why would he be looking for me after all these years? I realised it had required thoughtful planning and perseverance for Peter to find me across the world.

I phoned and spoke to Ian, Peter's carer. I remembered Peter as an athlete, fit and happy after exercise. The news of Peter as a quadriplegic was devastating. I could not imagine him losing the ability to move, what must have felt to him the essence of his existence. But life holds surprises and sometimes they must seem unacceptable, unthinkable.

Soon after I was told this shocking news I was able to phone Peter. It was so hard, he could not talk, I could only hear him breathing over the phone. What I said I don't remember. I was trapped between clouds and fog. We were miles and miles apart but yet I felt so close to him, like an immersion of heart and soul from a time long past. I was travelling back in time and I was 23 again.

Soon after this a letter arrived, then another, and another. It was inevitable, I had to go and see him. In May I jumped on a plane for Adelaide.

This next part of the story I choose to leave out. If anyone reading this has ever had an out-of-body experience and for the following days felt physically sick, they will know what I mean. It was just too painful and no words will ever come close to the feelings that took over. I looked into his eyes, held him tight and told him 'I am here'.

The days that followed were incredibly unreal. One day

Peter's carer had an argument with Peter and left him in his room, with only me to care for him. I knew nothing about caring for a person with such high dependency needs and I was terrified. Somehow under Peter's instruction we made it.

I remained in Adelaide for a few months. I wanted to give our relationship a chance but it was too hard, and with great pain in my heart I decided to return to my life in Rome. After just a few days I was back to the routines of my old life. But it didn't last very long. I knew something had changed. Something was missing, something that I needed in order to go on living. I needed Peter in my life. So I left Italy again, farewelled my family, friends and all those common places

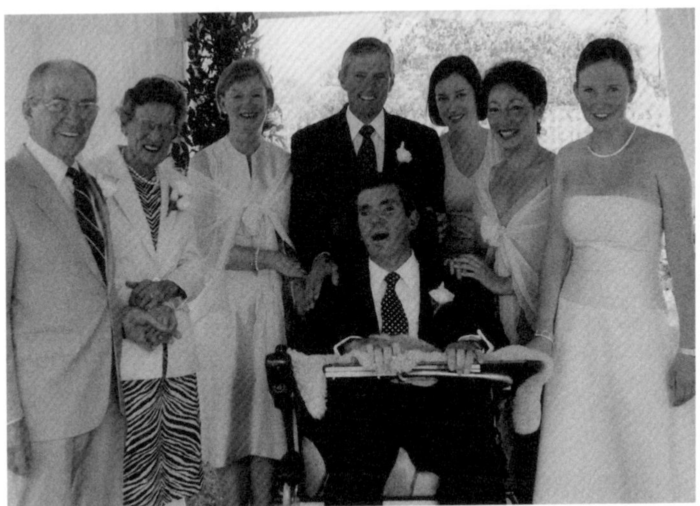

Our wedding day, 5 January, 2002

that were dear to my heart and flew back to Adelaide to start a new chapter of my life. And on 5 January 2002 in a beautiful garden, on a wonderful and unforgettable day, we were married.

Some lives are very complicated and are touched in ways that others may never know. I don't have the answers to any of this; I stopped asking and learned to accept.

Chapter 13

Life with Simona

Once my day started with the pain of flesh on flesh and my wait, in the early morning gloom, for the night staff to move me. Now my day begins in my new home in a tree-lined street at 6.45 am when I am awoken by my wife. She enters from her bedroom which adjoins mine so that she can hear me if I need help during the night. In the interests of a better and deeper sleep it was decided that separate rooms were wise. We commence limb-stretching exercises, always a relief after spending all night without movement. The radio switches on about now, to the station of my choice, providing the information for the current newsletter. Simona then sits me up and administers vitamins and supplements via the peg in my stomach. She cleans my teeth, ensuring my head is not tilted even slightly backwards because the toothpaste (which really burns) can run directly into my lungs, setting off a coughing spasm which has been known to last for hours. I am connected via my peg to a plastic bottle hung from a drip stand for my first feed for the day and then I await the arrival of the carer. During this time I will listen to the news on the radio, while Simona eats breakfast.

At 7.45 the morning carer arrives. I am shaved, then lifted by an electrical lifter into a shower chair with wheels. After my carer has showered me I am dressed, always in a jacket, ready for work. At 9.15 I am lifted from the bed to the wheelchair and I am mobile again. I am then taken out to my van, and driven to work. Once I am in my office and seated behind my desk I can express myself. I can write letters, pay bills, work on my newsletter or book, or otherwise engage in all the details of life. I regard the production of *Hermes*, the monthly newsletter, as being of critical importance to my general mental health and well-being. It keeps me alert, interested and keen. Usually, I am awake by 3 am and so my head has been at work for seven hours, thinking and planning, before I start in the office.

Jan de Palma, a registered nurse, has been employed for over seven years as my secretary. She is integral to my working day, attaching my feed line twice each day, making me laugh, and doing the 1001 little things necessary to keep me and the office running smoothly, and leaving me free to focus on my writing. I know that I can be difficult sometimes, but I seem to be forgiven this as we swing into each new day. The common thread is that literally every five minutes is important if I am to get all my work done on time. Jan understands this, therefore I am fed and medicated regularly. She blesses me with a routine, care and humour.

I began writing by using a thumb switch, a plastic splint fitted to my arm, to activate a computer programme. Initially this was painfully slow, but I improved to the point where I could use my index finger, which was vastly quicker, and allowed me, for example, to write several letters a day, to publish my monthly newsletter and, after persisting for

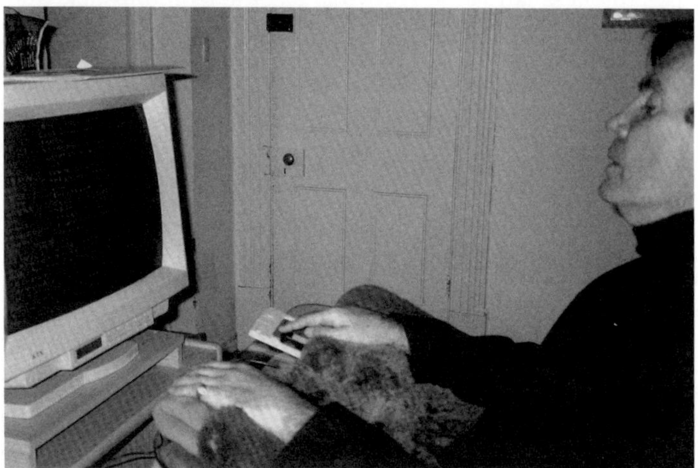

Recording my story on the computer using single-switch operation, at the office, Adelaide, 2005

13 years, to write this book. It is amazing the speed which can be reached with years of practice. It provided me with the opportunity to achieve something with this second life. I operate the computer with a single switch pad and use the Words Plus programme. The computer represents a form of freedom for me. I can construct my sentences any way I choose. Long passages of prose if I desire, complete with punctuation. Once again I have a measure of control over what is happening around me and I have access to the cleansing purity of work.

I have a rigorous exercise therapy session every Monday and Friday for about two hours, split between the arm pulley machine and the leg standing frame. One of the best exercises involves Ian hooking my hands onto a broom stick, and standing astride me. He is strong enough to lift my torso from the floor. I do about 30 of these, exercising muscles which are otherwise difficult to reach when sitting in a wheelchair. Every Tuesday, Wednesday and Thursday I have a soft exercise therapy session. This may also last for two hours and includes percussion (slapping of both sides of the lungs) which prevents the deadly sticky mucus from adhering to the bronchial walls. If I feel poorly, I might only exercise for an hour or so. After two hours (I wish there were more hours in the day to do more) I am wheeled back to my post in front of the computer. Between repetitions of a given

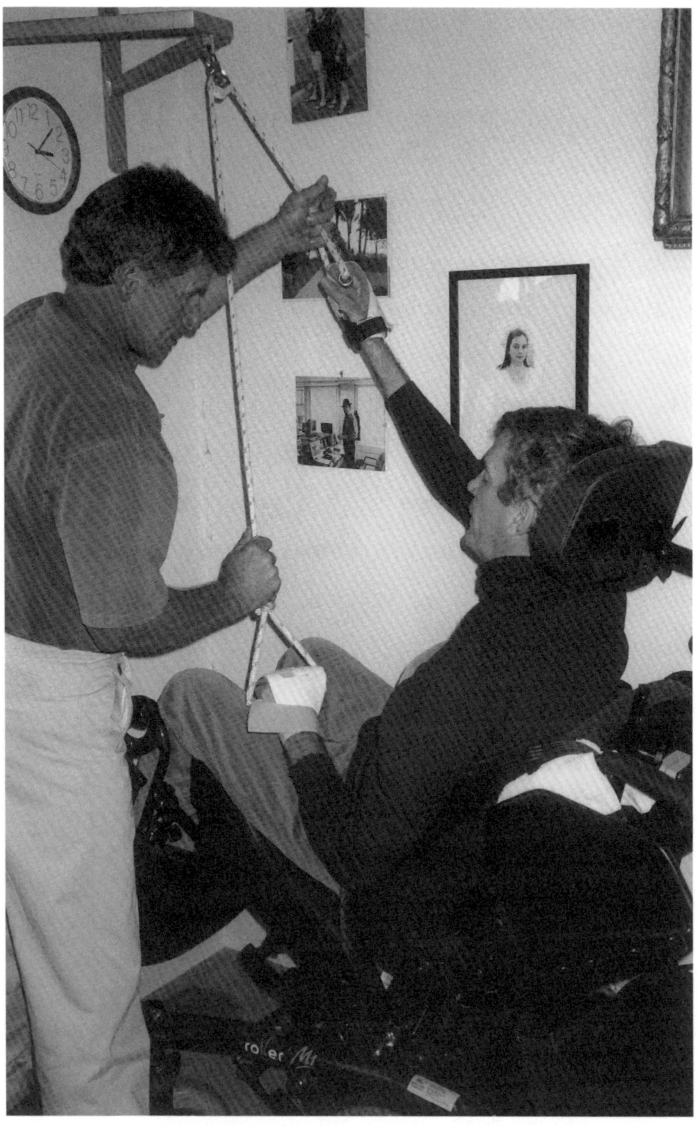

In the office physio room with Ian using the pulley machine, Adelaide, 2006

exercise or whenever there is a timely pause, Ian reads to me from the daily press, keeping me abreast of current events. And on Saturday mornings, a charming lady called Lorraine reads to me from 10 till 1.30 pm.

At 5.30 I am collected by Simona and we make the short drive home. Once there I will either sit outside in the garden (if it is warm) for about an hour, or watch the evening news on TV, or just be done with it all and watch some cartoons. The evening carer arrives at 6.15 and, with Simona's help, toilets, washes, strips me of my day-time clothes, and lifts me into bed. My teeth are cleaned, I am propped up in bed (because I have no muscle control, this needs to be centimetre perfect and often involves a lot of fiddling about, pushing and yanking) and left in peace to watch TV. Evening vitamins are administered, my peg is cleaned and dried and I am given fresh juice (prepared by my dear wife). Even though I can't taste it, I anticipate this, my only intake of fresh food, keenly.

Simona connects my evening feed at 8.30 and between 10.00 and 11.00 settles me for the night by administering a couple of sleeping tablets in liquid form via the peg. She then places me in a foetal position, on my side, with a bottle in place, a pillow between my knees, and several pillows jammed into my back. This is not just for comfort during the night. They also stop me from falling backwards out of bed.

Positioning is vital. I need about ten pillows, and at no point can I have one bit of flesh touching or resting upon another.

Lastly, Simona attaches a little bell (arguably the most important thing of all in the struggle to avoid constant supervision) which I use to call for assistance, when necessary. This forearm splint, a device designed by Technical Aid for the Disabled, has a small doorbell switch attached with double-sided Velcro and allows me complete freedom at night.

We have replicated a hospital environment at home. There is no reason, other than fear, to remain locked away in a hospital. I have some control of my eyelids and one finger and I lead a more-or-less normal life.

Chapter 14

Rebecca's story

We were living in England. It was the Christmas holidays, 1992, and we had returned home from a family holiday in Australia, and a stop-over in Singapore to spend time with Mum's family. I remember being called downstairs in our house in London by Dad and Mum for an impromptu family meeting. These were rare so I knew it must be something serious. Dad explained that we would be moving to Singapore in a couple of months, and that he was leaving in a couple of weeks. A school had been selected by my parents whilst we were visiting Singapore and we should start preparing for the move immediately.

I was 14, the oldest of the family, and nothing short of furious. I was horrified that my parents had selected a school for us (me) without letting us (me) visit the schools whilst we were in Singapore a couple of weeks earlier. Worse still, it was the school my cousin had attended, and completely hated. The idea of leaving all my friends and going to some horrific international school brought an Oscar-worthy teenage angst performance. I refused to speak to my parents, unless completely necessary. I was terribly upset, and refused to go and deliberately failed the school entrance exam.

Dad left for Singapore. I was still not really speaking to them (when I could remember to keep up the bad mood) which has an unpleasant sense of irony given that I would never again have the chance to have a real conversation with Dad.

Everything changed on Valentine's Day. It started like every other one. Dad arranged for all of his girls (me, Mum, Sarah and Sophie) to receive beautiful cards from 'a secret admirer'. (He still does this today.) After that things moved quickly. My uncle Greg who lived in Singapore phoned to speak to Mum, which was weird. Our nanny Justine asked me if Mum had mentioned anything to me. I asked her what about, and there was no reply.

Mum became quite frantic that day. Eventually she told me that Dad had collapsed. She was scared and kept using the word 'crisis'. All we knew was that Dad couldn't talk and no one knew why. There were words being thrown around like 'stroke', 'MS', 'brain infection', 'poison'.

Mum flew to Singapore that night. She told us she felt better knowing she was going to be there soon. When something went wrong someone had always told us it would be okay. This time no one did. I knew this wasn't good.

Mum was away in Singapore for about three weeks. During that time, my two younger sisters and I were looked after by Justine, and a constant cavalcade of cousins and family friends dropping in with food and comforting smiles. Information about Dad's condition slowly filtered through. He couldn't talk any more, but I remember thinking that surely this wouldn't last. Never for a moment did I picture him as a quadriplegic.

When Mum returned from Singapore with Dad, the first thing I noticed was she had lost a lot of weight. Mum's story about the flight back was horrific. Dad nearly died and she was taunted by drunken soccer fans. It was a complete nightmare. The situation was escalating to major panic and I felt there was no one in control.

It was a Saturday and a lot of the cousins had come around. Everyone got quite boozed and Mum was distraught. I remember her saying that her life had fallen apart and she was dancing through what was left. She pulled me aside and gave me a choice. She explained we could either remember Dad as he was, or see him one last time. I cannot imagine the courage needed to say that to your daughter. The doctors told Mum that Dad had contracted pneumonia and could have as little as three weeks to live. I had been dreading seeing Dad and I hadn't expected to be offered a choice. I entertained the idea of never seeing him again for about ten seconds but then announced loudly that I wanted to see him. I also decided there was no way Dad was going to die; what was this, a joke?

When we arrived at the hospital we were taken into a waiting room where a doctor in his twenties who didn't look much older than me, asked us to sit down and warned us that Dad looked different. The doctor explained that Dad could still hear and see us and that his mind was the same. He then said, 'Sometimes doctors are able to make people better, and sometimes they aren't. But then, sometimes, people get better all by themselves.' I loved the doctor for saying that and went first to see Dad.

I walked to the intensive care ward and was ushered towards Dad's room. I looked in and the first thing I saw was a grey plastic device slipped over his index finger. I burst into weird uncontrollable tears and two remarkably tiny nurses – they came up to my elbows – cooed lots of 'It's okay, you poor love, you're okay . . .' And it helped. I pulled myself together, walked in, and it *was* okay.

Dad was in a wheelchair and had lost a lot of weight. He was barely recognisable. Mum was in there smiling. Getting used to talking to Dad without a reply was tricky at first, and I remember thinking that I made a dick of myself talking so quickly and saying so much rubbish. I told some terrible jokes to try and make myself more comfortable, but it was really hard. He looked so different; the muscles in his face were slack and wasted but his eyes were the same.

The next time I saw Dad, Mum was devastated. She had asked my cousin to drive us to the hospital to visit Dad who was really sick again. In those days, Mum was at the hospital every day. I didn't want to go. I pretended to be asleep in the car to avoid it. Things were bad; Mum was always so sad and there just didn't seem to be any light at the end of the tunnel. I wanted to just close my eyes and escape for a while. Seems that I wasn't the only one who thought that was a good idea. When we got to see Dad, he was doing the same. He had his eyes closed but we could see them flickering . . . he was awake. It was too much for him and we didn't stay long.

Dad survived those three weeks and was moved out of ICU into a public ward. There were all sorts of people in there: an old man, an Indian woman, most of them with head injuries and diminished mental function. Visits took on a whole new asylum feel. I remember meeting a man in a wheelchair who had a head injury as a result of a motorbike accident. My mum introduced us and he asked me how I was. I replied I was well and asked him the same. He responded, 'Well, I have good days and bad days, and that's how it goes.' It scared me to think that this was Dad's outlook now.

In those days Dad would need suction, a painful process where the nurses stuck a tube down through his tracheostomy tube and sucked all the gunk out of his lungs. It could make him go into convulsions and was quite horrifying. It was also terribly awkward; we never knew where to look. We wouldn't want to leave the room because that would look like we were uncomfortable (and it was all about being strong), but at the same time, it was so humiliating for Dad.

I remember feeling an overwhelming sense of sadness when I was told that it was unlikely that Dad was ever going to be like he was before his stroke. Not so much for me, but for Sophie. She was only three, and it was likely that she would never remember Dad as he was.

Dad came back to the house in London for a visit before we left. He had to be driven in a private ambulance, and for some reason I can't remember he couldn't come through the front door. At the end of our back yard there was a large communal garden, like a big private park, reserved for the tenants of the two streets that backed on to it. Dad had to come in through the garden gate on a stretcher which was quite bizarre and caused a commotion amongst our neighbours. He stayed for a while and I remember being upset when he left because the neighbours all stared so much. I knew they couldn't help it but I found it so offensive. I would eventually get used to the face you can't miss – a six-foot lanky guy in a monster truck-sized wheelchair.

Moving back to Australia was okay for us. Both Sarah and I had always felt an affinity with Australia. Even so, Julia Farr Centre was the furthest from ultra-cool London you could get. It was several storeys of concrete, gloomy, painted all shades of brown, and possibly the ugliest building ever built. I can never understand why these places filled with sadness have to look depressing too.

We visited Dad there after school, which was hard. The fact it was hard, made it harder, if that makes sense. It was the guilt. I hated that I hated going to see Dad there, but the place was terrible: the noises of the patients, the nurses who were sometimes friendly, sometimes not, the gloom and the smell. And I thought, if I hate this, imagine how Dad is feeling.

Both before and after his accident, Dad cut a strict figure in the parenting department. As is typical of Dad post-stroke, a wheelchair was not going to get in the way of whatever it was he had to do, disciplining children included. I think Dad's scolding was more powerful after his stroke. There was something really unnerving about having to write down your own telling off. 'You have really disappointed me ... How dare you talk to your mother ...' have an extra stinging edge when spelt out letter by letter.

As was the case in London, Dad was in the same ward as the head injury patients, because he has a similar physical presentation. We knew Dad's thinking was fine and it was hard listening to the painful wailing of those whose minds had gone elsewhere. Dad, having a peculiar sense of humour, had a joke about this: what's the difference between KFC, and JFC (Julia Farr Centre)? KFC provides the chicken, JFC the veggies. Not particularly fair, but then nor is waking up and being unable to walk or talk anymore ...

Since then, much has happened. I think a lot of families could have responded to this situation by being scarred and damaged. I remember Mum saying once that she wanted to make sure that we, the children, came out of it all as unscarred as possible. I feel confident that we have all become stronger as a result of our experience, which is a credit to Mum and Dad's parenting skills, both as a team and independently. Dad has come a long way. He got out of

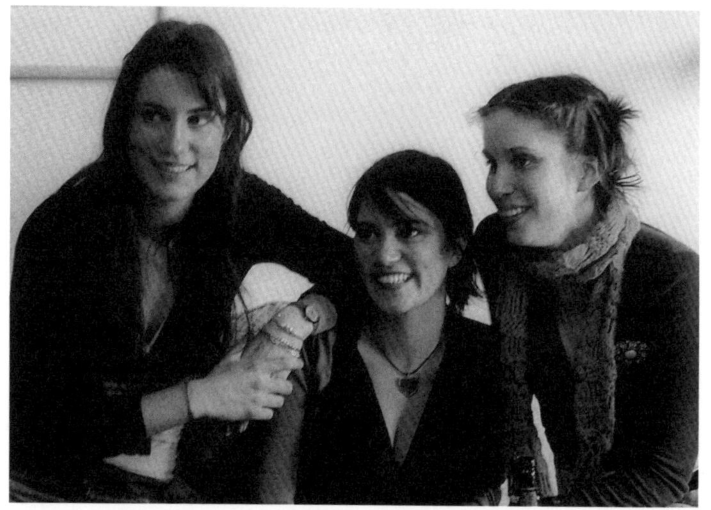

My three daughters: Sophie, Rebecca and Sarah, 2005

JFC and runs a business with his newsletter. He tracked down and married Simona and bought a house. I am proud of him.

Chapter 15

The Hardest Thing of All

I realise there are many things that I can't do (like eat fresh crispy bread, go for a run, play the piano, lie on the beach in the sun after a good bodysurf, hold my wife or my children) but I try not to think of them.

Fortunately there are tracts of my face which are not paralysed, but my tongue and throat muscles don't function well enough to allow me to swallow safely, and my right eye is basically useless. My left eye, out of which I obtain most of my vision, has a marked ocular bob, making reading difficult.

The deficiency which irks me the most is my inability to eat. After all I can compensate, to some degree, for each of the other skills destroyed by my stroke: I use either my eyes or the computer to communicate, I use the physiotherapy sessions to satisfy my need to move, and I use my jerky bouncy left eye to see. These are not perfect solutions (few things in life are), but they will do until something better comes along. For *eating* however, I have no compensation, no substitute.

I am 'fed' four times a day via a small plastic gastrostomy peg in my stomach. If I did not have this peg, I would have to take my meals orally, which would mean a significant portion would go directly into my lungs and I would either choke to death or drown – slowly. I had already been to hospital more than once, on the first occasion with both lungs collapsed, following one stint of overly ambitious (on my part) oral feeding.

So at feeding times, rather than grieve, I simply put on a different head and I am elsewhere. Before my stroke, I treated every meal as a small banquet. I would never eat while on the move, or while standing up. Food and the ritual of eating were serious and deserved to be celebrated.

There is no point inflicting pain on myself by reminiscing on the lost joys of eating; the rush of a creamy chilled beer or the yeasty warmth of fresh bread. To dwell on what I have lost increases my anguish, makes each day a little harder. So I use thought control to travel to other places and I avoid the destinations of my past which cause pain or sadness. In my mind I can go anywhere. I can focus on the important things –

things that I can do something about. I used to get distressed about not walking; I longed to walk, to feel the easy swinging rhythm as I covered ground. Now I don't; I accept there is nothing I can do about it. Instead I can concentrate on staying alive long enough for advancements in medical science to return me to some of the pleasures of my lost life.

I have changed a great deal over the past few years, not in the trite way of simply becoming more patient or more tolerant, but in the more complex matter of 'getting a life'. Not being a believer in re-incarnation or other such mystical beliefs, I reasoned that this was the only life I had and that I had better get on with it. At the start of every day, we can each choose to be happy or sad, that choice is entirely our own. But the former is far more conducive to healing than the latter (plus one looks upon each day more positively), so for me this was not a very difficult decision to make. This is not one of life's difficult choices.

I lived my first life like a tornado and now, in my second, I am to 'reap the whirlwind'. I was almost 42 when I suffered the stroke and I knew what kind of person I was. I had lived intensely, grabbing life's opportunities. Whatever this next life holds in store, I am not going to spend it wishing 'if only I had . . .'

And I have been given a chance. If I had been born at any other time, I would not have survived my stroke. I emerged unable to move anything except my eyes, but I am alive. I can laugh, and most important of all, I can think. Economic and political conditions are good. I haven't endured a depression or a major war, and modern engineering means that both my vehicle and my wheelchair allow me mobility. Technology (and eye movement) provide me with the means to communicate.

But I have to maintain my rage; to guard against that 'oh well' feeling that comes with time, and brings with it a sense of security in the present. I must continue to rage against the status quo (wheel chair and all) for there is real danger in making life too comfortable, and forgetting old challenges and the joy of achievement.

The hardest thing of all, when totally bestilled, is to maintain dignity, a sense of self-purpose and masculinity. The only solution can be to adopt the appropriate mental stance, much of life is lived in the head anyway. For me, this process of living life in my head has become a constant, a way of life; *every* waking moment is spent this way. And by wearing the 'right head' it is possible to continue. In short, to be more or less convinced that life is 'normal' is the only way I have found to claw back some of the dignity that had been lost.

Chapter 16

The Final Step

At last, the nightmare may be over. I am now carrying (I hope) a full dose of umbilical-cord stem cells which will continue to multiply within my body. It is my fervent hope also, that stem cells will be to the 21st century what antibiotics were to the 20th century (causing many pharmaceutical companies to suffer a sharp decline in both sales and profits). The following story took nearly six months to unfold and probably wouldn't have happened at all without the organisational skills and sheer persistence of Simona.

On Monday 27 December 2005, Simona and I came to my office to tidy a few loose ends. An e-mail had arrived from the UK from my one-time work colleague – and now firm friend – Andrew. In it he detailed the work of Dr Robert

Trossel of the PMC Clinic in Rotterdam, Netherlands. Andy had suffered from severe multiple sclerosis for several years and had flown to Rotterdam for treatment and was glowing in his praise. This message from Andrew was like manna from heaven for us, filling us both with immediate, and much-needed, hope. My father had always said that a cure would be out there somewhere, if only I could manage to stick around – and maybe here it was! There followed a flurry of messages and faxes between the UK and Adelaide which convinced us that we had to give stem cell therapy a go. From the start I felt supremely optimistic about the possible outcome.

For those thinking that flying to Rotterdam for therapy was a relatively easy task, please think again. Every possible step presented a hurdle. In order to qualify for acceptance for this treatment, I needed to have several things done. My peg (gastrostomy button used for feeding directly into my stomach) needed to be changed. Although unpleasant, this proved to be relatively straightforward. My blood test needed to show no signs of infection. Again, no problem; the results came back clear. I needed to remove all mercury from my system. In particular this meant removing all the old amalgam dental fillings from boyhood, and replacing them with porcelain. For reasons of haste, and because a specialist was required to do this work, I booked in to the South Australian dental hospital. A preliminary appointment or two were necessary in order to decide how best to proceed. Then, after several rather nerve-wracking decision changes about whether to take out certain teeth or leave them (and therefore risk infection while we were away), the decision was finally made to leave them alone and just remove the amalgams. The dreaded day of the procedure eventually arrived. It had been decided that this could all be done in day surgery rather than being admitted to the hospital overnight. I was relieved to hear this as I imagine the inside of a dental hospital is not particularly cheery. So far, so good – no teeth had to be whipped out, and no overnight stay.

The day was windy, overcast and grey (which pretty much matched my mood). Simona and I waited in a vast, rather grubby, waiting room. This area was mostly quiet, with the background noise of people muttering, and the intermittent, not-so-comforting whine of the dentist's drill. Suddenly, there came a loud, blood-curdling scream – from the room I was about to enter! The waiting throng erupted into laughter, and someone said what everyone else was thinking: 'Well, that sure helps the confidence!' Despite my misgivings, the two-hour procedure went smoothly, a tribute to the skill of the dentist involved.

In order to get a ticket to Rotterdam, I needed to have a current passport (my old one had expired years before), and in order to do that, I had to have a series of passport-sized photos taken and signed, as to true likeness, always with a form of some kind. Maddening and time-consuming but unfortunately necessary. And patiently and efficiently my dear Simona organised everything and bore the anxiety of another task to be done.

We also thought it appropriate to seek a second opinion. This was a complete flop. The neurologist we met completely discounted the likelihood that what we were about to do could possibly have a favorable outcome. In his opinion, this was all hippie-style nonsense, probably done with 'smoke and mirrors', and when asked if he would undertake the procedure himself, he flatly replied 'no'. This did not exactly fill us with confidence but we now felt that there was an irresistable force pushing us forward, towards Rotterdam.

In case you are thinking that only the rich could afford such a treatment, this certainly wasn't our position. The treatment cost around AU$20,000, but I needed to travel with two carers, so all the travelling and accommodation costs had to be multilplied by four. In short, around AU$50,000 and a huge amount of effort (mainly by Simona) was invested in this little 'shot in the dark'. To readily gain access to this rather princely sum (which I didn't happen to have just idly sitting around) we decided to extend our mortgage. At this juncture, all roads definitely pointed to Rotterdam!

Occasionally I suffered a fall in spirits and I would recall my father's advice to 'keep on keeping on' because a cure was out there somewhere. To get some idea of just how low I would get sometimes, try as you are reading this, to sit perfectly still without fidgeting or changing your position in any way, without moving a muscle, eating a thing, or uttering a sound – for five minutes. This was my position permanently! All year, every year.

So of course I was very keen (desperate even?) to try this new treatment. But by God, it was hard going. Everything needed to be booked (and in some cases paid for) in advance: liquid food for me (now in plastic bottles because aluminium cans are thought to be potentially harmful), a lifter, slings, a shower-chair, hotel rooms, Access cabs, medications, and so on. And all this had to be arranged in a different time zone; for us this meant working largely at night.

We were required to pay for this treatment in advance, which meant taking a leap of faith and sending a considerable sum of money into the ether, to an organisation which may, or may not, exist, for an, as yet, medically unproven technology. To make matters worse, every attempt we made (whether by e-mail, fax, or phone) to contact the office manager of this company, was met with total silence. At this point, our frustration and apprehension was eased somewhat by further news from Andrew that all was well, and that he was making good progress following his own treatment.

An even more frustrating incident occurred the weekend immediately prior to our departure. On the Friday evening (when it was too late to cancel our flight tickets), we received a telephone call – a recorded message no less – from Rotterdam saying that there was a chance the stem cells were not available! What did this mean? At this point, we were like a heavily laden plane gathering speed as it lumbers down the runway for take off. So much effort and planning, we just couldn't stop now! But this was a potentially devastating problem. An e-mail was sent to the company immediately, and we both spent a sombre, depressed weekend.

As we prepared to depart for the airport very early on that chill June Monday morning, Trossel himself replied encouraging us to make the journey and assuring us that the stem cells would be available. As I waited outside in the early morning semi-darkness for Simona to lock up the house, I reflected on what lay ahead, and the huge gamble we were taking. For all that, I remained supremely optimistic of a favorable outcome. The reply from Dr Trossel ensured that we would make the trip across with a lightened heart.

The trip to Rotterdam was pretty uneventful. Simona had pre-measured my feeds, and the water which followed, and put them into a refrigerated carry case and taken it on board. I was fed during the flight as usual, but instead of hooking the bag up to a feedstand, Simona hooked it on the luggage compartment and then jammed it shut.

For those who are unfortunately wheelchair-bound but who still nurse a desire to travel, I would suggest at least doubling your normal water intake (and avoid putting booze into the bottle) and taking a roho cushion for your bottom. I find this essential. To avoid slipping off your chair, and to avoid an uncomfortable bow in your back, place the roho about eight centimetres from the back of the chair. Also take on board a eucalyptus inhaler. The air on board is pressurised and very drying (hence the added water), bloody cold (so put away your Hawiian shirt and thongs), and recirculated (so if the guy up the back has a cold . . . look out!). The steam of the inhaler will help keep your lungs clear, while the eucalyptus oil will help disinfect them. I used mine about every three hours with the assistance of the hostesses providing a small quantity of boiling water.

So we made it to Amsterdam. Moreover, when we arrived at the airport, not only did my wheelchair and all its electrical parts survive the trip well, and re-assemble without drama, but also our taxi driver (arranged months beforehand) was there on time for the final leg to Rotterdam. This part of the journey was largely conducted in silence, as we sped along the Dutch freeways in the very early morning.

The hotel in Rotterdam was a huge disappointment. We entered a cold, musty, only partially lit foyer, with windows that looked as though they hadn't been cleaned in years. Worse was to follow. We caught the lift up to our floor, which was immediately distinguished by the smell of stale tobacco smoke, and after a short walk down a stuffy, dimly lit corridor warm air. After indignant calls to management demanding we be moved, we learnt the hotel was booked solid – as indeed was every other hotel in town. This was not what we had booked, but there wasn't a lot we could do about it!

The equipment which we had hired was also faulty, but we were advised that it was all that was available. Later that day Simona went to the PMC clinic to ensure that we would get the stem cells as promised. We had been travelling for 34 hours, and we all needed a rest. We were exhausted and disappointed but we had arrived.

I was totally focused on getting those stem cells into me (that, after all, was why we had travelled so far), which probably didn't make me the ideal travelling companion. Until that happened, I couldn't really pay much attention to anything else. The next day, we had a compulsory booking at the Aqua Tellis Centre about two hours away. This involved my wife and I completely naked (so far, so good) taking a bath with 100 per cent humidity designed to make the body sweat out any impurities. Well, I hardly perspired at all, I mean really hardly a drip! This indicated my dietary intake was almost perfectly balanced. I use a product called Jevity, which precludes me from building muscle-fibre, but which nourishes me sufficiently to allow me to complete all my physical exercises every day, plus the (sometimes quite heavy) mental work-load associated with running the business. Also it meant that after innumerable permutations and combinations, I had probably struck the right balance between physical and mental exercise, and the right type of exercises to ensure that each major muscle-group received attention. The Aqua Tellis procedure took most of the day. Suitably cleansed, we were now ready for the big day.

The injection of stem cells (1.5 million umbilical-cord cells, gathered and frozen in Switzerland) was carried out by Dr Trossel himself, in the hygienic premises of the PMC clinic. I did not have to go into hospital for this. Rather it was all done in the clinic with me sitting in an armchair. Quite simply, I was given an injection of placenta in the thigh, followed about an hour later by the stem cells delivered into me by an intravenous drip in my wrist, and by three jabs in my neck and four around my navel. All quite painless. Now I had to keep as well as possible because an

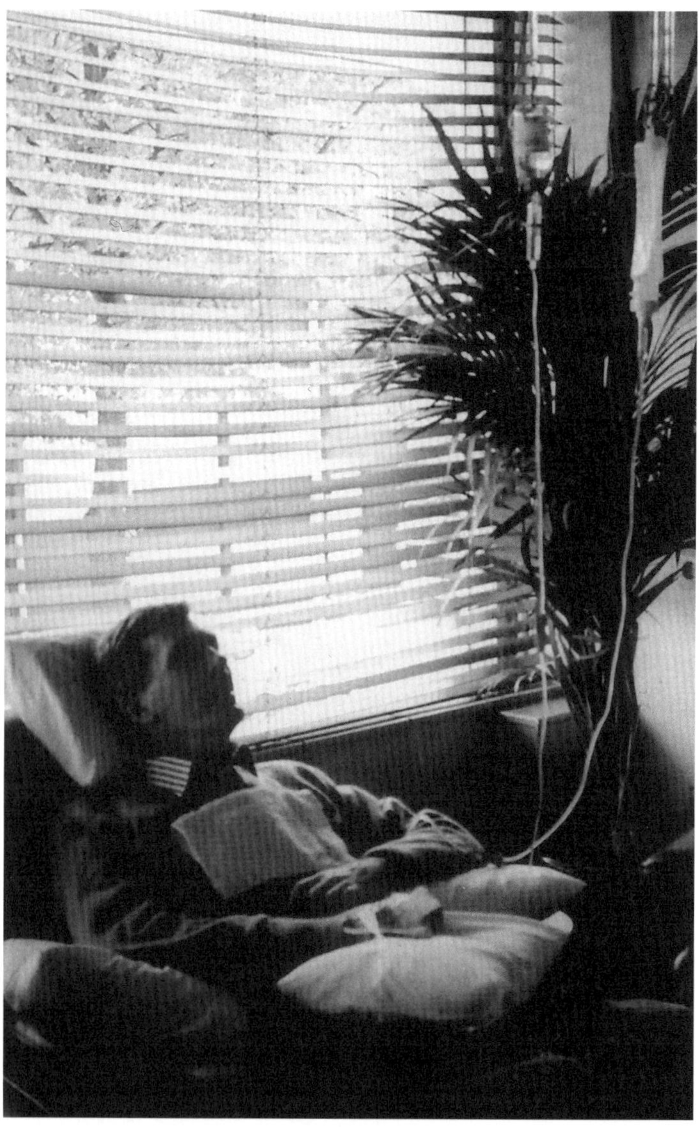

Receiving pre-treatment before stem cells, PMC Clinic, Rotterdam, 8 June, 2006

infection is thought to damage, or even kill, stem cells, and just wait. I felt a bit like a portable incubator.

The process was over by lunch-time, leaving the rest of the day free. On the weekend my old friend Andrew and his lovely wife Gillian came over from the UK. I was particularly pleased to see them, and we spent a brief but pleasant time with them. On the Monday we completed another Aqua Tellis treatment, and it was time to fly home.

The flight out may have been uneventful, but this was a nightmare from beginning to end! Everything that could go wrong, did go wrong, due mainly to the fact that the airline staff were simply unaccustomed to, and unprepared for, dealing with a person in my position. I felt like some sort of museum exhibit, tied up like a sausage with my knees nearly touching my chin, perched precariously on one of those impossibly small airline chairs, and being whizzed from terminal to terminal at a rate of knots. It was only luck which prevented a foot or a leg from snagging on something. I now permanently have a titanium rod in my left leg courtesy of many breaks from just this type of accident. At one point, all the ancilliary airline staff lined up to stare at the 'elephant man' as I motored through. Pity I wasn't carrying a little flag to wave as I went past! Perhaps needless to say, our little party was delighted to hear that our aircraft had begun its descent to Adelaide.

Epilogue

We had been told it would take three to six months for the stem cells to start having an effect. And three months after the treatment in Rotterdam, almost to the day, I began to notice changes. At first it was a strengthening of my limbs, then improved flexibility in my fingers, particularly in my left – the worst – hand. I noticed I could suddenly bend the top joint on my left index finger. And the left side of my face (previously frozen into a sort of hitched-up position so when I smiled it was a lop-sided grimace), now slid into place after 14 years. But the most significant improvement occurred to my swallowing. First I noticed I could handle my toothpaste water without choking, then I developed a desire to taste Simona's cooking, and, after assessment by a speech pathologist, I felt confident I could risk eating again. For the first time in many years, I could look tomorrow square in the face and know, without doubt, that I would be in a better position than today. I knew my obstacles but the passage back seemed clear. Knowledge replaced blind optimism.

Cared for by Simona, I felt I was in the best physical condition since the stroke. But weak! My hands and wrists were small, fine and pale, like porcelain. I barely recognised them as my own. I redoubled my daily physio intake – not more or even longer sessions but increased effort with every exercise – and spent more time in hydrotherapy. And six months after the treatment I made decisions to change my life. I needed more time and energy to concentrate on advancing the effectiveness of the stem-cell treatment. I closed the office and ceased writing the monthly newsletter. Writing an accurate and up-to-date newsletter each month had exhausted me to my limit. Running the office had been important. It had given me a way back into the real world, I had contributed to society rather than be a drain on it, and it had woken my brain, forcing me to think again. But it was also hideously expensive and it was exhausting. Its time had passed.

I began to feel stronger and my muscle memory improved. This meant when I stepped up the exercises I believed my muscles would store the knowledge they had gleaned. I progressively lowered the handle bars on the standing frame and loosened the belt around my chest. This meant when I stood I relied less on the hydraulic lift of the machine and more on the power in my arms and legs. The increased strain was enormous and I brought an extra shirt to work, so profusely did I sweat during these sessions. I was fortunate every muscle, every sinew, every bone held through this process, because a break or a tear would have been disastrous.

The progress continued. I can now flex my muscles at will. Every morning in the shower I work at moving my torso from side to side. I can direct the shower head to wash myself and can briefly sit unsupported. I never tire of rediscovering the inside of my mouth, sending my tongue on exploratory missions around my teeth. I can eat a 200 gram pot of yoghurt and a 150 gram pot of vitamised fruit with ease. Gradually this process of waking my body will, I know, lead me to the Holy Grail. I will rise from this damn wheelchair and walk. Who knows, I may even be able to talk.

In addition to teaching me to slow down – life doesn't have to be lived at a thousand miles an hour – my stroke has taught me to cherish my family, my mother and father, my brother and his wife and children, and of course my own dear children; and Simona, my precious wife. Without their devotion and 'never give up' attitude, I doubt I would have made it. I am 57 years old and I have Simona. I have so much to look forward to and so many things still to achieve and I am growing stronger every day.

Of all the qualities with which I have had to arm myself, patience, persistence and a positive attitude have been the most important – they are such precious qualities. And so is laughter, the life-giving power of laughter. These are my lifelines.

For Dad, Christmas 2004

Toe tapping in his armchair, an embracing splendour
Ready to marvel in my world.
Perched faithfully on his knee
Absorbs tears of a stairwell confession.
His hands in mine hold me tight
As I soar in flight around him.
Cobbled country pathway bike rides
Paving our bramble bush journey together.

Yet sweet splendour suffocated by fate's cruel hand.
Now motionless body taunts his sharp mind.
But I see you still, love divine
You shine more radiant despite the darkness.
Memories are these that frame my love.
He carries me through what life's made of.

Sarah Couche

Wakefield Press is an independent publishing and distribution company based in Adelaide, South Australia.

We love good stories and publish beautiful books.

To see our full range of titles, please visit our website at www.wakefieldpress.com.au.